THE FASTING FACTS

A BOOK FOR MEN AND WOMEN THAT TOUCHES ON INTERMITTENT FASTING, THE BENEFITS OF FASTING, HOW TO FAST FOR BEGINNERS, AND HOW TO BURN FAT THROUGH FASTING.

D.J. PREJEAN

CONTENTS

INTRODUCTION: WHAT MAKES FASTING DIFFERENT?

You have tried them all and nothing works, you always end up right back where you started or even heavier. All we have to do is look around us to see that diets, exercise, medication, surgeries, do not work to sustain weight loss. Why? Because they are not sustainable, we go into these with the best of intentions, yet we fail. Is it us, or the system? Let's take a look at the common diets of the past and why they didn't work for you.

Dieting is a billion dollar industry. While people do lose weight dieting, they do not retain that loss. As soon as they achieve their goal, their diet is over and they start eating like they were before they lost the weight. Even how we look at the word 'diet' is an issue. Oxford Language defines diet as, "the kinds of food that a person, animal, or community habitually eats" (google.com). The key word being habitual;

meaning constantly. Whatever we did to get to our goal, we need to continue. That is why most diets fail, we see them as temporary, not constant. Dieting restricts your eating, makes you feel like something is being taken from you. You begin to resent the fact that the food is there but you are not allowed to eat it. So, once you reach your goal, you see yourself as being free of these restrictions and you go back to the way you ate before.

THE OBESITY EPIDEMIC

Before we can try to understand dieting, we need to understand how we got to this point in time when being overweight has become the focus of much of the world. The current condition of our weight has become a worldwide epidemic. Obesity has become a worldwide crisis. This was not always the case; in fact, it is fairly new.

Only in the last few decades, since the {eighteenth} century, has our outlook on food changed. With advances in agricultural technology, we began the transition from scarcity to abundance. At the beginning, this was a good thing. Healthy food was available for all classes, and we began living longer and healthier lives. To look at this from a nutritional perspective, it was quite simple; we began to take in more energy than what our bodies needed. Our bodies, in turn, took that extra energy and stored it as fat for times of food scarcity, which were now few and far between. In the past, one of the greatest exertions in mankind's life was the procurement of food (Eknoyan, 2006).

However, as technology continued to advance we also saw a change in the type of food being produced and how we lived our daily lives. We became a society of eating and leisure in abundance. At the time, this was seen as a positive. Society had been plagued by the issue of food scarcity and malnutrition for so long that having extra body weight was seen as a good thing, especially in women. Even as men's bodies took on a lean, more muscular form, women with extra body weight were still viewed as desirable. In the medical world, it was still recommended that you always carry a few extra pounds, as it was believed that your body would need to rely on this during a time of illness. Doctors were advising patients to gain weight, not lose it (Eknoyan, 2006)!

By the nineteenth century, however, our opinions of weight and physical size began to change. Being overweight was no longer the desired look and the impact of it on our physical well being became a query within the medical world. The first group of doctors to publicly promote the negative image of being overweight were psychiatrists, identifying two well known eating disorders of anorexia nervosa and bulimia. Over eating went from being seen as the result of depression or hypochondria, to being a result of our own undisciplined behavior, to being a psychological disorder. By the mid 1900s, the study of fat gained speed, with it being classified as its own organ with its own hormones and cellular bodies. Once it was recognized in this manner, the study into fat and its properties was recognized as a worthy pursuit. The connection of a person's weight, particularly obesity, has been a focus of many studies and scientific research since this point in time (Eknoyan, 2006).

There are many obesity related health problems in today's societies, worldwide. Obesity is determined by one's body mass index (BMI). Your BMI is your weight in kilograms divided by the square of your height in meters. You are considered overweight if your BMI is over 25, and obese if over 30. One of the first diseases to be associated with obesity was diabetes. Diabetes occurs when the levels of blood sugar in your body cannot be regulated either because your pancreas cannot produce enough insulin, you are insulin resistant, or both. Almost 17 million people in the U.S have type 2 diabetes. Of those, 67% have a BMI of over 27, and 64% have a BMI of over 30 (Related Conditions, n.d.).

High blood pressure is when your blood pressure goes over 140/90 on a regular basis. About one out of five U.S. adults have high blood pressure, with men being more likely to be affected than women, and African Americans twice as likely as Caucasians. Of those with high blood pressure, the statistics are as follows: in men, 47.1% have a BMI between 25 and 30, and 60.4% of women have a BMI between 25 and 30 (Related Conditions, n.d.).

Cancer is the uncontrolled growth of abnormal cells from healthy cells. These abnormal cells prevent the proper functioning of our organs and damage the essential systems of our bodies. Recent studies have shown that the death rates from cancer were 52% higher for men and 62% higher for women with a BMI of more than 40. One study indicated that women who gain more than 20 pounds from the ages of 18 to midlife, have double the chance of developing breast cancer (Related Conditions, n.d.).

High Cholesterol is also a growing problem in our society. High cholesterol is a lipid disorder caused by a high level of fatty substances in your blood. These substances include cholesterol. Among those in the U.S. diagnosed with high cholesterol, 40.7% of men have a BMI between 25 and 30, and 60.1% of women have a BMI between 25 and 30 (Related Conditions, n.d.).

Other health complications related to obesity are heartburn, gallbladder disease, osteoarthritis, sleep apnea, stroke, heart disease, and psychological depression. We will discuss some of these conditions and the positive effects fasting can have on them, as well look at the short term and long term benefits of fasting (Related Conditions, n.d.).

COMMON APPROACHES TO DIETING

Many people feel confused about where to start when it comes to dieting, so they often join an organized weight control group, such as Weight Watchers. These diet groups often teach nutrition, offer group support, and a weight maintenance regime. While success can be achieved with these programs, the long term weight loss is minimal, and the programs can become expensive over the long haul.

Formula diets involve taking in the minimum amount of required nutrients in liquid form. Many of these plans consist of liquid or powder supplements to be taken one to four times a day, some allowing for one meal a day. Slim Fast and Cambridge Diet are examples of this type of program. The advantage of these programs is that there is little decision making and they can be convenient. However, they can be costly, teach nothing about nutrition, and can be very unhealthy if used for an extended period (Dieting, Nutrition, Britannica, 2019).

Low-carbohydrate, high-fat, and high-protein, which promote ketosis, have grown in popularity. On this diet, sugars and starches are restricted and meat, fish, and cheese intakes are increased. Although calories are not counted, this change in macronutrient intake will lead to a decrease in consumed calories. This reduction in calories, along with the ketosis process, will result in weight loss, quite rapidly at first. However, once normal eating habits are reintroduced, the weight comes back. Also, prolonged adherence to this diet method is not advised, as it can have dangerous effects related to the secretion of uric acid (Dieting, Nutrition, Britannica, 2019).

High-carbohydrates and high-fiber diets promote eating mainly whole grains, vegetables, fruits, and nuts. While high-fiber foods do make you feel full and have fewer calories than most foods, they are bulking agents; they are indigestible. They promise slow weight loss, if you also exercise and consider the nutritional makeup of your food. This diet requires a fair amount of thought and effort, for little gain. As well, some are so low in calories, protein, or fat that they may be unsafe (Dieting, Nutrition, Britannica, 2019).

Diet aids come in pill form, and they claim to either suppress your appetite or reduce your stomach space. Some of these diet pills are amphetamines, starch blockers, benzocaine, diuretics, and thyroid hormones. While amphetamines can be highly addictive, with dangerous side effects, other ingredients have proven to have no effect on weight loss (Dieting, Nutrition, Britannica, 2019).

Exercise is also a proven way to lose weight. It's simple; burn more calories than you consume, and you will lose weight. However, exercise requires time and endurance. We all live busy lives, and it is quite easy to come up with an excuse not to exercise - too busy, other obligations, too tired, etc. This can become a bigger problem for those who start exercising with great enthusiasm, and adjust their diets to support their new activity level. When they stop their physical routine, they often continue to eat as though they are working out and actually gain weight (McKnight, 2018).

Surgery is the last resort for many, and it is effective at the beginning. Like any weight loss method, however, bariatric surgery requires a lifestyle change. Immediately after surgery, you can only eat small amounts of food, and you are required to exercise. After awhile, your stomach will begin to stretch, especially if you constantly eat until you are full. With overeating comes the lack of desire to exercise. So, your meals get larger and you move less. You end up right back where you started, consuming more calories than you are burning; the result, weight gain (McKnight, 2018).

BEFORE YOU START ANY WEIGHT LOSS PROGRAM

No matter what the reason is for your consideration to start a weight loss program, whether it is simply to lose weight or to improve your health, there are several things you need to consider. First of all, do not feel like you have to do it all on your own. Tell your family and close friends. They can be a great support system, and may even want to join you.

There are three important components to consider in weight loss -- your weight, your Body Mass Index (BMI), and your waist circumference. Most people simply focus on the number on the weight scale, but that is not a good indicator of your health or your risk of weight related diseases. Your BMI and waist circumference are better tools to use. Your body mass index or BMI is the main factor your doctor will use to determine your health risks. {Your BMI is determined by your weight and height, specifically; your weight in kg divided by your height in meters squared.} If you have a BMI index of 20-30 you are considered overweight. If you have a BMI of over 30, you are considered obese. There are many BMI calculators on the internet (What You Should, 2020).

The most dangerous type of body fat is that which collects around your waist. To get your waist circumference, place a flexible tape measure at the top of your hip bones and around your body until it meets. It should not be tight, but should not be able to slip down either. If you are a woman and your waist circumference is greater than 35, or a man and your waist circumference is greater than 40, it is considered to be unhealthy (What You Should, 2020).

So what makes fasting different from any other weight loss method you have tried in the past? Every diet method above talked about calories. There is no reduction of calories in fasting; you simply change the time of day you consume these calories. You change one thing about your day, but you change nothing about your diet. Fasting is a lifestyle, not a diet.

1

THE HISTORY & SCIENCE BEHIND FASTING

HISTORY OF FASTING

There are records of ancient peoples and civilizations fasting. The act of fasting was a pillar of many religions and ethnic groups. Many people believed that the gods would not speak to you until you had fasted for an appropriate amount of time. Other cultures used fasting as a means of penance for the sins you had committed. If your crops failed, you fasted. Not out of necessity, but to appease the angered god so that he would be more generous the following harvest season. With the Native Americans, fasting was always, and still remains, to be a vital component of several of their traditional ceremonies, such as the vision quest. Shamans often directed people to fast as a way to heal unknown illnesses (Fasting, 2021).

Fasting continues to be part of many major religions today. Some Buddhist monks use fasting as part of their meditation practices, and followers of Jainism use fasting as part of a practice to achieve a transcendent state. Many Western religions practice, or at least encourage, fasting during certain religious periods, such as Yom Kippur, Advent, Lent, and Ramadan (Fasting, 2021).

Fasting has been used as a form of protest to express social and political views. Perhaps the most well known individual to practice fasting as a form of protest was Mahatma Gandhi. His fasting as a means of nonviolent protest caught the attention and support of the entire world. Fasting has been used in the past century as part of protests against the treatment of Black Americans, Native Americans, Irish Nationalists, and many more (Fasting, 2021).

Medical fasting has been used since the 5th century BCE, when physicians recommended it to patients with certain illnesses. Through watching the natural instinct of humans and animals to turn away from food during illnesses, it became an accepted belief that not only could fasting help with the healing process, to not fast may be detrimental to the body healing (Fasting, 2021).

By the late 1800s, great advancements were made in the understanding of the physiological effects of fasting. By the 1900s, fasting was being used in clinics and hospitals to treat or prevent certain illnesses. Some fasting methods, particularly those for chronic diseases, consisted of more than a month of dry fasting, followed by a period of consuming only water or calorie liquids, as well as exercise and enemas. Other modified fasting treatments allowed for small amounts of daily calories (200-500), along with physiological or religious therapies. The allowed calories had to be from particular foods, such as bread, vegetable broth, etc. Lastly came the introduction to intermittent fasting as a means of treating and preventing certain diseases (Fasting, 2021).

SCIENCE OF FASTING

Before you can understand the science behind fasting, you have to understand the science behind food. People generally believe that protein is good, and that fats and carbohydrates are bad. This is not the case. Each food has its benefits and its potential dangers for our bodies. The food we eat falls into one of three macronutrients:

- Protein
- Carbohydrates
- Fat

Protein is considered to be the building blocks of cells. It is involved in the building of cells, the transportation of oxygen through our bodies, immune function, and skin elasticity. So, as you can see, protein is essential. While protein comes from many sources, animal protein is the best. But, not in the form of red meat, as this often contains a lot of saturated fat, which can be unhealthy. While animal meat is considered complete protein, it may be more 'complete' than you bargained for. Many animals raised for food today are injected with antibiotics and hormones, the effects of which on humans is still unknown. Vegetarian food contains incomplete protein, so you need to be sure that you eat a variety of vegetables containing different kinds of proteins. Of course, it is always best to choose healthy proteins in high quantities. This can be found in fish, eggs, and soy (McKnight, 2018).

Carbohydrates have gotten a bad rep during recent years, especially in the diet world. Carbohydrates are essential to your life. They are the direct source of energy that your body needs in order to function. Without carbohydrates, you would constantly feel worn down as your body would be working double time to get the energy it needs to keep working. However, there are different types of carbohydrates; some are bad and some are good. You should not avoid all carbohydrates, as besides being the body's main source of energy, they contain micronutrients and minerals your body also needs to stay healthy, but make sure you choose the right ones (McKnight, 2018).

Good carbohydrates are also complex carbohydrates. These take time for your body to digest and are good for your body. Complex carbs would be found in foods like, millets and barely, breads, cereals, and oats, to name a few. Bad carbohydrates are also known as simple carbohydrates. Your body can use them instantly, and they increase your blood sugar. These carbs increase your food cravings and cause you to gain weight quickly. Processed foods, fast foods, sugar and artificial sweeteners, chips, cookies, and alcohol are just some of the commonly consumed foods that are bad carbo-hydrates (McKnight, 2018).

Fats were perceived to be the cause of weight issues and other health problems long before carbohydrates were. This aversion to fat may be even more dangerous than that of carbs. Most people still buy low fat or nonfat foods, even if they avoid simple carbs. What they don't realize is that these foods usually replace the fat with sugar or artificial sugar, which has been proven to be worse for you than the fat that was removed!

As protein is the building blocks of cells, fats are the building blocks of hormones, which are the body's communication medium. As with other macronutrients, fats come in both bad and good forms. Unsaturated fats are known as healthy fats. These are found in fish, nuts, and olives. While satu-rated fats, found in butter, cheese, cake, etc. are also needed by the body, they are only needed in small quantities. So these saturated fats should not be consumed in large quantities, as that will be harmful to your body.

Scientific studies of fasting diets for the purpose of losing weight began over 100 years ago in lab animals. When calories were reduced by 20-40%, the animals would live longer and had a lower chance of chronic illness and disease. In 2008, the first clinical trial on calorie reduction, called Calerie, was conducted. After two years and only reducing their calorie intake by 12%, most participants saw a drop in blood pressure, cholesterol, glucose, and insulin. The people following the Calorie reduction experiment had aged slower than the control group. However, there were negative side effects noted as well -- trouble sleeping, reduced libido, low energy and hunger. Some participants were removed from the study for safety concerns, such as loss of bone density and lean body mass, and for losing too much weight (Barna, 2019).

Our body is preprogrammed to shut off when calories are reduced, which activates genes that tell its cells to preserve resources. Cells no longer grow or divide, but stall, making them more resistant to disease and stress. Enter a process called autophagy, where dead or toxic cell matter is cleaned out, and damaged cell components are repaired and recycled (Barna, 2019).

Recent studies have shown that genetics, the amount of carbs, proteins, and fats, as well as regular exercise, also play a factor in the effectiveness of calorie reduction. These findings, combined with what was found in the Calerie Trial, and the unlikelihood of extensive reduction of calories, the idea of reducing calories for only a certain time period, or fasting, was born (Barna, 2019).

In order to understand the current trend towards fasting and why it has been proven to be a superior way to lose weight, we need to examine the first attempt to formalize a method of weight loss, calorie restriction.

CALORIE RESTRICTION

A calorie is used to measure the amount of energy contained in a food source. In 1918, a nutritional text was published that promoted counting calories and calorie reduction as a method to lose weight. This book, *Diet & Health: With Key to the Calories* simplified the concept of calories, so that it moved from the scientific world to the common household. The author of the book, Lulu Hunt Peters, even went so far as to encourage people to refer to their food, not by its traditional name but by the calories it had (Heffernan, 2016)!

Peters, who struggled with weight herself, went into the psychology behind the struggle many people experience, such as not having a supportive partner or peer group. She also talked about roadblocks, such as cravings that we all encounter. For example, the only food she promoted as an absolute to avoid, was candy. That was due to her opinion that it was too easy to eat too much of, not because of its sugar content. In fact, her guideline to lose weight was simply to eat 1,200 calories a day, and you would lose weight. There was no thought to what macronutrient group these calories would come from. You could eat whatever you wanted, except candy, as long as you stayed at this calorie limit. The formula Peters used to come up with a more personal calorie reduction diet was if you wanted to lose weight; multiply your body weight by 15-20, then eat 200-1000 calories less than that number. If you wanted to gain weight; you ate 200-1000 calories more (Heffernan, 2016).

There is no doubt that calorie reduction does help to lose weight. This method of dieting has been around for over 100 years. It's quite simple to back, if you eat less calories than you need, your body will turn to stored energy for fuel, and you will lose weight. If you eat more calories than what you need, your body will store these excess calories as fat, thus you will gain weight. But does this mean that calorie restriction is the easiest, most efficient or healthiest way to lose fat?

We have learned through the years that knowing how many calories to eat each day is not as simple as multiplying your body weight by 15-20 and eating 200-1000 calories less. There are many more factors involved -- your gender, age, physical activity levels. You need to know how many calories your body needs to function during the day and eat less than that amount. With the invention of technology, there are many programs out there today that will give you an estimate of what your body burns in a day. There are also several great programs out there today that you can use to fit the calorie content of your food (Heffernan, 2016).

One major issue with counting calories today, is that food portions continue to increase. Restaurants are especially deceptive in this area as a single serving on the menu can actually be 2-3 times more than what a single person should be eating. In order to count calories accurately, you need to know what a true portion actually looks like. Here are some handy ways, according to West, to measure your food when you do not have scales or measuring cups handy (2016).

- 1 serving (½ cup) rice or pasta=rounded handful or computer mouse
- 1 serving of meat (3 oz.) =deck of playing cards
- 1 serving of fish (3 oz.)=checkbook
- 1 serving of cheese (1.5 oz)=tube of lipstick or your thumb

- 1 serving of fruit (½ cup)=tennis ball
- 1 serving of green leafy vegetables (1 cup)=baseball
- 1 serving of vegetables (½ cup)=computer mouse
- 1 tsp of oil=fingertip
- 2 tbsp peanut butter=ping pong ball

Even these measurements are much easier to use for some foods than others. For example, how would you figure out the calories of a slice of pizza? Counting calories can be hard and frustrating, which is one of the reasons why people find it hard to stick with.

In recent years, there has been more of a focus on what you eat as well. This is where one can see the faults in simple calorie counting and restriction. Not all foods with a caloric count of 100 will be equal. Different foods have different effects on hunger, appetites, and how your body burns those calories, which in return affects our energy levels, moods, susceptibility to disease, etc. Even counting calories, you need to be eating high quality, nutritionally dense foods. So overall, while counting calories is a good practice, it will be most effective if you combine it with other dieting strategies, such as macronutrient portion control and intermittent fasting (West, 2016).

KETOSIS & KETONES

Another important body function one must understand to comprehend the benefits of fasting is the process of ketosis. When we eat, especially carbohydrates, our body has a readily available source of glucose. Glucose is the fuel our bodies use for energy. In today's society, we often eat too much, and our body will store the energy, or glucose, that it does not need in the body, for when it is needed. If we take away that food source, the body uses the glucose and fat stored in our body as fuel. Fatty acids go to the liver and are oxidized, where they produce ketones (Richter, 2020).

Ketones are essentially molecules made from fatty acids, which are created when the body is going through a period of low blood glucose levels. While we normally have small levels of ketones in our bodies, once we start fasting, the brain sends a message to the liver telling it to produce mass amounts of ketones. There are three types of ketones: acetone, acetoacetate, and beta-hydroxybutyrate (Richter, 2020).

These three ketone types are transported around the body by the blood and can easily cross the blood-brain barrier. So, not only do these ketones provide energy to the body in the absence of glucose, they are a great source of energy for your brain as well. Ketones will continue to rise up to ten days after you begin to fast, this is why people often report feeling energized after their first two or three weeks of fasting. Many also report having better concentration, clarity, and mental energy. So, not only can fasting lead to medical benefits like burning body fat, it can also improve brain function as well (Richter, 2020).

2

TYPES OF FASTING

By the early 2000s, studies were showing positive results of fasting. There are many different approaches to fasting, whether it be only eating during certain hours of the day or fasting only 2 days out of the week. While many people believe that fasting means no calories at all, only water, this is not the case with most fasting diets. You are allowed non-caloric drinks and sometimes calories on fasting days, but a very limited amount, and only from certain foods. If you google fasting, intermittent fasting, or even intermittent fasting for weight loss, you will get hundreds, if not thousands of search results. This can be so overwhelming that you may just give up and stick to your current diet. Hopefully, the information here will clear up some of the confusion and allow you to pick the fasting diet that would be best for your lifestyle (7 Different types, 2018).

WATER FASTING

As the name suggests, this fast involves drinking only water for a certain amount of time, usually 24-72 hours. Water fasting has proven to have some benefits besides being a quick way to lose weight or detoxing. It may help fight off chronic disease and break down damaged cells. Some studies have even shown that it can lower the risk of certain types of cancers. There have been several modifications to the water fast that allows you to add certain no calorie or low caloric items to your water, such as lemon or cucumber. However, it can pose a lot of risks, and is not easy and can be risky if followed for an extended time (Raman, 2017).

Prior to starting a water fast, you may want to prepare your body by cutting back on meals and introducing more water into your day. While on a water fast, most people will drink two to three liters of water a day. During this time you may feel dizzy, so you may have to alter your regular activities. After your fasting days, you still have to be very cognizant of what you eat. Do not eat a big meal, as this will cause a lot of discomfort. Start with smaller meals or easily digestible meals several times a day (Raman, 2017).

Studies have shown that water fasting may help break down and recycle damaged cells in your body. It is believed that when damaged cells accumulate in the body, we become more susceptible to cancer. The recycling of these damaged cells can also help prevent Alzheimer's and heart disease, as well as prolong your life. Longer water fasts should always be done under medical supervision. Longer fasts have been shown to have lowered blood pressure (Raman, 2017).

There are several risks and dangers associated with water fasting. The first is the type of weight you lose. You will lose weight quickly on a water fast, but it is not the type of weight that is beneficial to lose. This weight loss will most likely come from water, carbohydrates, and muscle mass, not from fat cells. Ironically, a water fast may lead to dehydration. A lot of water we get comes from the foods we eat, when we cut out these foods, we need to make sure we compensate through the water we drink. The bottom line is to drink a lot of water when on a water fast. A lot of people experience a sudden drop in blood pressure when water fasting. This can cause dizziness, lightheadedness and even fainting. All of these side effects can be dangerous in the wrong situation, therefore you may need to adjust your daily activities. Gout, diabetes, and eating disorders may all see a rise in symptoms during a water fast. As with any diet, if you have any of these diseases, do not water fast without speaking to your doctor first (Raman, 2017).

JUICE FASTING

Juice fasting has been around as long as any type of fasting; it was even mentioned in the bible. In 1920, Dr. Max Gerson created a diet for health purposes based on organic fruit and vegetable juice. Also known as juice cleansing or detoxing, this diet promotes only drinking the juice of fruits and vegetables for a certain period of time, typically three to ten days. There are several ways to complete a juice fast -- drinking only juice and water, drinking juices with dietary supplements, combining juices with colon cleansing proce-dures, and drinking juices while on other specific weight loss diets (The Full History, 2017).

No matter which approach you take to juice fasting, there are three important stages to follow. Begin preparation three to five days before you begin, gradually eliminate certain foods such as coffee, sugar, meat, dairy, wheat, alcohol, and nicotine. This should reduce headaches, cravings, and other withdrawal symptoms while you begin your fast. You should also increase your intake of fresh vegetables, fruits, and fluids. During the cleanse itself, which will last one to three days, you will drink at least 32 ozs. of juice or smoothies, with half of that being green vegetable juice. After the fast, it is recommended to eat only small, light meals and take several days to gradually add food back into your diet (Wong, 2021).

There are some benefits to fruits and vegetables, as they are high in vitamins and minerals which could boost our overall health. Juices are high in anti-inflammatories, which may boost our immune systems and give us more energy. Juices may also improve digestion and flush toxins out of our bodies. While advocates of the juice fasting claim these are some of the benefits of following their cleanse, there is no scientific evidence to back their claims. In fact, doctors have identified potential risks of juice detoxing (Withworth, 2018).

Drinking large amounts of juices may be harmful to some, especially those prone to kidney disorders. Many juices contain an acid called oxalate, which contributes to kidney stones and other kidney problems. Juice can stimulate your bowels, causing you to lose too many nutrients and experience dehydration. Juicing fruits and vegetables yourself may contaminate your food. You may be skipping a vital step, such as pasteurization, or other procedures to remove bacteria, which in return may make you sick. You may experience a drop in your blood pressure, causing dizziness, lightheadedness and even fainting. All of which can interfere with your daily activities and safety. Lastly, while you will lose weight, it will not be a lasting weight loss, as it will not target your fat cells, but will mainly be a loss of water weight and muscle mass (Withworth, 2018).

DETOX DIETS

Detox Diets are a type of fasting diet which leads people to believe it has a cleansing or purifying effect by using the word detox. These diets may help your body get rid of the chemicals and toxins we absorb in our day-to-day lives. The problem is that "cleansing" is arbitrary work and it is almost impossible to measure. We know that the liver is the "cleansing" organ of our bodies, and that fasting does release and breakdown the stored glucose in the liver, that it lowers triglycerides and raises HDL levels. These are signs that the liver is moving fatty acids back into the liver for processing and eliminating (Oberg, n.d.).

As part of the detox diet, participants replace one or two meals a day with an organic, pea based protein smoothie. They also eat a full meal of lean protein, vegetables, and healthy fats. This is supplemented with extra fiber, water, and milk thistle. Also of equal importance, you cannot have sugar, alcohol, caffeine, gluten, red meat, or dairy (Oberg, n.d.).

DRY FASTING

When you dry fast, you take in no food or water for a certain period of time. The thought behind it is that when you dry fast, your body will use stored food and water during this time. The results found with dry fasting were pretty much the same as intermittent fasting. As a result of a dry fast, you can expect to lose weight, lower blood pressure, reduce body fat and inflammation, repair and regenerate damaged cells, and fight premature aging. It also promotes brain functions and emotional benefits by clearing your mind and energizing your spirit. There are several different ways to do dry fasting, intermittent, prolonged, and absolute (Greenleatherr, 2019).

With intermittent dry fasting, there is a set time frame for eating and fasting during the day. This is the method most supported by the experts, as you get a chance to refuel your body before you enter a period of dry fasting. On this diet, it is up to you when you fast and when you eat. Common time frames are 16:8 - 16 hours of dry fast, followed by an 8 hour window to eat, or 20:4 - dry fast for 20 hours and your eating window is 4 hours (Greenleatherr, 2019).

Prolonged dry fasting, involves going without food and water for longer than 24 hours. This approach is not recommended like the intermittent dry fast is. The human body is made up of 70-75% water; therefore water is a vital component. Going without water for more than 24 hours can do more harm to your body than good. Your organs need water to function properly, depriving them of water can cause irreversible damage (Greenleatherr, 2019).

Absolute dry fasting is the most extreme. You do not have any contact with water whatsoever. You do not brush your teeth with water, wash, or bath! There is no evidence to support absolute dry fasts to have any health benefits to intermittent dry fasts. Dry fasts appear to have more spiritual backing than scientific.

If you would like to try dry fasting, follow these recommendations:

- Ask yourself if this is the right fasting method for you. With little to no added benefits between dry fasting and fasting that allows water, you must keep in mind the added risks.
- Prepare your body. A few days or even weeks before you start a dry fast be sure to eat enough healthy fats -- avocado, fatty fish, and nuts -- to sustain your body's needs. Also, cut caffeine out of your diet. This will help with withdrawal symptoms.
- Water fast first. You should only try a dry fast after you have tried fasting which allows water for a few weeks.
- Increase your fat intake. This is mentioned above, but this recommendation refers specifically to the last meal you eat before your fast. A meal high in healthy fat, (a ketogenic meal friendly meal would

be the best) will reduce discomfort at the beginning of your dry fast.

- Stick to your schedule. For best results, stick to your fasting schedule. If you try dry fasting and like it, stick to the same schedule if you want to repeat or extend your dry fast.

Ultimately, dry fasting is not for everyone, but you will not know if it is for you if you don't try it. With the little or no extra benefits between water fasting and dry fasting and the dangers that could result, it may be best to stick to a fasting method which allows you to drink water.

FAST MIMICKING

This type of diet is more of a combination of calorie restriction and fasting. On this diet, one eats very small amounts over a certain period of time, usually five days. These foods are usually high in fat and low in protein and carbohydrates. While you eat often, you are not consuming many calories, and many people find the low caloric intake to be hard to follow with this diet. You will lose weight on this diet, just from the reduction in calories, but you will also receive many of the benefits you get from restricted time fasting (Shortsleeve, 2020).

This is the macronutrient breakdown of this diet. Day one: 11 percent protein, 46 percent fat, and 43 percent carbs. For the next four days: 9 percent protein, 44 percent fat, and 47 percent carb. Also important is water intake, two to three liters a day. You can exercise on this diet; low to moderate intensity only. Intense exercise and heavy lifting should be avoided. If you find it difficult to keep track of your macronutrients, you can always sign up to a food service which will follow this diet for you (Shortsleeve, 2020).

Let's take a closer look at this diet. This is not a diet you do on your own. You have to buy their food. When you sign up and pay, you will receive five boxes of prepackaged food to be eating in a particular order. During those five days, you eat only what is in the kit; soups, crackers, drinks, supplements, etc. You are also encouraged to drink water and decaffeinated tea. These foods make up a low carbohydrate, high protein, high fat diet, that is very low in calories; 1,1000 the first day and 750 for each of the next four days. This is not enough calories and, if followed for an extended period, would lead to health issues. The program itself recommends doing it under the supervision of a medical professional and to avoid exercise during the five days that you eat their food. The program recommends that you follow it from one month to six. That can become very costly. Each month's shipment of food costs 249$US (Kubala, 2019).

ONE MEAL A DAY (OMAD) DIET

This is an extreme fasting diet, where you only eat one meal a day. So, basically you fast for 23 hours a day, then you eat one big meal of whatever you want during a one hour period. While this diet does not dictate what or when to eat, it does recommend that you eat after your most active time of the day and you eat only healthy food. There can be clinical benefits to the OMAD diet. If your weight loss stalls on intermittent fasting, OMAD method can jump start your weight loss. Results indicate that this method of intermittent fasting can speed up the benefits of other methods. This could be beneficial for people who live very busy lives, but little research has been done into this diet (Scher, 2021).

As this is a method of fasting, it should have some of the same benefits, such as stabilizing insulin levels, decreasing blood pressure, and improving metabolic syndrome, among others. If widening the fasting window can help improve these conditions, then OMAD should do so!

There are some concerns over the OMAD method, however. If you have a history of eating disorders, you should not try this method. Only being able to eat for one hour may trigger bingeing. If you use this method for a long time, you risk not getting enough calories to remain healthy. Long term calorie restriction will actually decrease your metabolism, which is the opposite of what you want for weight loss. Because you are only eating one meal a day, you will not be able to eat enough protein. Protein is very filling, so it is hard to eat a lot of protein in one sitting and still get enough of the other macronutrients you need, as well. These other macronutrients are easier to consume, and as a result we may end up with a protein deficit. As we know, protein is a major building block for cells and not getting an adequate amount of protein can lead to a variety of health issues (Scher, 2021).

Excessive carbohydrate intake can be an issue as well, especially for those who are insulin resistant. On the OMAD method, you need to have all your carbs in one meal, where normally those carbs would be divided into several meals. If you are highly insulin resistant, 20g of carbs in one sitting may lead to a rise in glucose and insulin levels, taking your body out of ketosis. Stomach upset and diarrhea is likely. When you go a long time without eating, it is a shock to your system to have to deal with food, especially if you overeat. If you take medication that should be taken with food more than once a day, check to see if other opinions are available. If you must take with food, then this is not the diet for you. If you follow a strenuous exercise routine, it could be dangerous to continue if you are on the OMAD diet. While mild exercise is always recommended while fasting, intense exercise is not (Scher, 2021).

KETOGENIC (KETO) DIET

This diet has gained great popularity in recent years, although there have been mixed results and mixed reviews. While it does not involve fasting, it is worthy to examine in a book about fasting facts, as its ultimate goal is to get your body in a state of ketosis. Fasting does the same thing.

The ketogenic diet focuses on the amount of macronutrients you consume. While there are different versions, they all follow the following general ratio: 60-70% carbs, 20-35% protein, and 5-10% carbohydrates as your daily macronutrient intake. This is promoted so that your body can enter a state of Ketosis. Ketosis is the process whereby your body starts to use stored glucose and fat, causing your liver to release ketones into the blood. This process is also achieved through fasting. In fact, it is achieved quicker through fasting, and there is no monitoring of your macronutrients. Actually, there are practitioners of the Keto diet that recommend you fast while on the Keto diet in order to achieve ketosis faster (Richter, 2020).

3

BENEFITS OF FASTING

F asting involves periods of normal eating followed by periods of fasting. There are many proven benefits to intermittent fasting. Some of them are clearly visible from the outside, shortly after we begin our new way of living. Others occur inside our bodies and are not so visible to others, but should be much more important to you. As you read through the short term benefits, you will notice the repetition of many scientific words and bodily processes. This is because the human body is a complex system where all components work together to allow us to function as we should. There is a huge overlap in certain hormones, proteins, cellular bodies, etc., that influence multiple functions of our body.

SHORT TERM BENEFITS

Short term benefits will be seen and felt fairly quickly after you begin intermittent fasting. Of course this depends on your commitment to the method and individual body composition. Not everyone will see the same results at the same time, but they will occur when the time is right for you.

Weight Loss

Probably the most common reason why people fast is to lose weight, especially if it is just five or ten pounds for a special occasion. In this case it could be a combination of just a reduction in calories, which would lead to weight loss over time, but fasting gives it a boost. Short term fasting will increase your metabolism as well, resulting in a higher weight loss. Studies have also shown that fasting can increase the level of body fat you burn as well, especially belly fat. Studies have shown that you can typically lose seven to eleven pounds over a ten week period. You may be tempted to fast longer to see if you can lose more weight but remember, if you want to lose weight in a healthy manner and keep it off, it is recommended that you only lose one to two pounds a week. According to Gunners, "short term fasting actually increases your metabolic rate by 13.6-14%...intermittent fasting can cause weight loss of 3-8% over

3-24 weeks...people also lost 4-7% of their waist circumference." As for muscle mass, traditional calorie reduction in people is 75% fat and 25% muscle mass; with fasting, it's 90% fat and only 10% muscle mass (Gunners, 2016)!

Human Growth Hormone

The human growth hormone (HGH) appears to be affected by fasting as well. The HGH is a protein hormone that is involved in regulating the body's growth, metabolism, weight loss, and muscle strength. It is believed that fasting increases the levels of HGH in your body. HGH is also affected by the body's levels of insulin and blood sugar, in that the more stable they are, the more HGH is optimized. According to Mawer, "one study found that 3 days into a fast, HGH levels increased by over 300%. After one week of fasting, they had increases to a massive 1,250%" (2019).

Autophagy

This is a process where damaged cells get recycled into new, healthier cells. Cells can only divide so many times, then they are programmed to die. However, autophagy kind of saves the cells from this fate by regenerating the damaged parts of the cells instead of allowing the whole cell to die. During this process, old cells are broken down into component amino acids, which are the building blocks of protein. When we fast, amino acid levels rise, and one of three things happen to them. They can go to the liver for gluconeogenesis, they can go through the tricarboxylic cycle and be broken down into glucose or they can be incorporated into new protein. So, what activates autophagy? Nutrient deprivation or fasting. So, by fasting we stimulate the removal of old, damaged proteins and cellular parts. Fasting also stimulates the human growth hormone, which tells the body to start producing new cells. What turns off autophagy? Eating. So, when we fast, we are basically putting our bodies through a recycling phase (Fung, 2016).

Blood Sugar and Insulin Levels

Fasting helps stabilize blood sugar and insulin levels in the body, both of which are critical in controlling diabetes. Fasting is an effective way for people with type 2 diabetes to reduce insulin resistance. This allows the body to more efficiently transport glucose from your bloodstream to your cells. This, combined with lower blood sugar levels, can prevent the spikes and crashes often experienced by people with type 2 diabetes. This control of insulin can also help lessen the symptoms of PCOS in women as well. In human studies on intermittent fasting, fasting blood sugar has been reduced by 3-6%, while fasting insulin has been reduced by 20-31% (Coyle, 2018).

Blood Pressure

High blood pressure is the most determining factor in whether a person will develop cardiovascular disease. The American Health Association has recently reclassified what constitutes hypertension (high blood pressure), creating three classifications. A stoic pressure of 120-129 and a diastolic of above 80 is considered elevated blood pressure. A stoic of 130-139 and diastolic from 80-89 is classified as stage one hypertension. Lastly, a stoic pressure greater than 140 and a diastolic pressure of more than 90 is stage two hypertension. Based on these new classifications, almost half of U.S. adults have high blood pressure (Understanding Blood Pressure, 2010).

The good news is, you do not always have to rely on medication to get your blood pressure under control. Elevated insulin levels can lead to the accumulation of salt and fluid in the blood, which can lead to high blood pressure. We have discussed above how fasting can stabilize insulin levels. Perhaps of greater importance is a protein known as the brain-derived neurotrophic factor (BDFN). This protein stimulates the release of acetylcholine, which affects blood pressure in two ways. First, it reduces your heart rate, and second, it expands blood vessels. These two changes combine to help lower blood pressure. Scientists believe that intermittent fasting increases the production of brain-derived neurotrophic factors (DeSantis, 2020).

Cholesterol

Cholesterol is a major risk factor for heart disease, yet it is totally treatable. Cholesterol is broken into two classifications: low density lipoprotein (LDL), or 'bad cholesterol; and high density lipoprotein (HDL), or 'good cholesterol'. Another blood component we look at when examining cholesterol is triglycerides. Triglycerides are a type of fat found in the blood, they move freely throughout our bodies, and they can be used as a form of energy. During fasting, triglycerides get broken down into fatty acids, which the body uses for energy, and glycerol. Cholesterol, on the other hand, is not used as a form of energy, but it is used in cell repair (Fung, 2016).

In the early 1960s, it was discovered that high cholesterol along with high triglycerides were associated with heart disease. At first, it was thought that we got high blood pressure from eating foods high in cholesterol; however, it was later discovered that 80% of the cholesterol in our blood is produced by our liver. Studies have shown that while eliminating fat or eating very low amounts, we can lower our cholesterol, but unfortunately, it lowers both our LDL and our HDL levels. We must remember that fats are an important macronutrient for other bodily functions, as well (Fung, 2016).

So, the ultimate question is how does fasting affect cholesterol? Studies have shown that fasting can lower our LDL cholesterol levels. One study showed that after 70 days of alternate daily fasting, LDL levels fell by 25%, and there was a 30% decrease in triglyceride levels. However, fasting appears to have little effect on HDL, which is a good thing (Fung, 2016).

Inflammation

Inflammation can make us feel hot and swollen. It can also lead to such conditions as heart disease, rheumatoid arthritis, multiple sclerosis, and cancer. Studies have shown that fasting can help decrease levels of inflammation and thus could prevent the development of these inflammatory diseases. Ghrelin, known as our 'hunger hormone', increases in those who intermittently fast. Ghrelin is also believed to have an anti-inflammatory role in our immune system. Inflammation contributes to weight gain, and weight gain causes inflammation. Therefore, if we decrease our weight through intermittent fasting, which is said to indirectly have an anti-inflammatory effect, intermittent fasting can help with chronic inflammation. Not only will you lessen your chances of developing a chronic inflammatory disease, you will also feel more comfortable, as well. There are several other hormones affected by intermittent fasting that deserve investigation. We will look more at fasting's impact on inflammation later when we discuss the long term benefits of fasting (Berger, 2019).

Cortisol and Adrenaline Levels

Cortisol and adrenaline are two hormones that work together to produce our 'fight or flight' responses. When you experience something you see as a threat, your hypothalamus, a tiny area at the base of your brain, sends an alarm to your body. This tells your adrenal gland to release cortisol and adrenaline. Adrenaline increases your blood pressure, your heart rate and your energy levels. Cortisol is your main stress hormone; intermittent fasting decreases your levels of cortisol. Therefore, when you fast intermittently, you can get the added adrenaline needed for increased energy levels, while lowering your stress levels. This could account for the increased energy and alertness people feel when fasting (Chronic Stress Puts, 2019).

Leptin Levels

Leptin is a hormone that is produced in adipose cells, where we store our fat. This hormone controls our hunger. When we reduce leptin and increase ghrelin, we activate our biological response to not having food. This signals the body to start using the stored fat. Once your body gets used to the fasting cycle, you won't feel the intense hunger you did earlier in your fasting. While there has been extensive research done on laboratory mice, no studies on the types of adipose cells have been conducted on humans. These laboratory results, however, have been promising (Newman, 2017).

We have two types of fat in our bodies, white and brown. White fat stores our excess fat and releases it when the body needs fuel. However, it is also the type of fat associated with type 2 diabetes and obesity. Brown fat on the other hand, burns energy and can positively impact type 2 diabetes and obesity. Under certain circumstances, white fat can become brown (in some cases, beige) fat. When the mice were put on an intermittent fasting diet, they had a lower percentage of white fat cells than the control group because they had converted to brown fat cells (Newman, 2017).

Stomach

Giving your stomach a break from digesting food can give it time to replenish good gut bacteria. Your stomach is very sensitive to food or the absence of food. When food is absent, there appears to be a significant increase in bacteria associated with positive health markers. These appear to be a constant cycle within your stomach and digestive system, when you are awake and eating, there are bacteria in your stomach associated with negative health markers. When you sleep and there is not food entering your stomach, there is a rise in the bacteria associated with positive health markers. So, when you fast and get food out of your system for a longer period, there will be a higher build of these positive bacterias in your stomach (Schwartz, 2020).

Mental Alertness and Memory

Many argue that fasting helps improve mental alertness. In laboratory animals, fasting has shown an increase in the production of BDNF, which we discussed earlier. This protein affects other components of the blood, as well. BDNF plays an important role in learning, memory and the generation of new cells, as well. Autophagy, as discussed earlier as well, is the regeneration of damaged cells, which is increased during fasting. Our brain, just like the rest of our body, is composed of cells, so this recycling of cells occurs in the brain as well. Old, damaged cells are repaired and function as new cells, resulting in better reasoning and mental alertness (Fung, 2016).

When the body is starved of carbohydrates, the brain triggers the liver to start releasing what is stored in the body. This process releases ketones into the body. Ketones can be used by some parts of the brain as a direct energy source, boosting its ability to learn and remember. It has been known for decades that these ketones are an effective method of controlling seizures in those with epilepsy. Improvements in spatial planning, working memory tasks, and on working memory capacity tests showed improvement after only four weeks of intermittent fasting. Research on animals has shown improvements in memory and learning (Richter, 2020).

Improves Mood

Research has shown that after three months of intermittent fasting, participants reported improved moods with decreased tension, anger and confusion. Another study showed that intermittent fasting had positive effects on emotional well-being and depression. Fasting can also stimulate the production of the neurotransmitter GABA, which stabilizes anxiety. Another theory is that a mildly negative stimulus (fasting) can protect against a subsequent more severe insult (depression). As well, fasting increases BDNF, thought to influence antidepressants, synaptic plasticity, the regeneration of new cells, and improved stress tolerance. One study of healthy volunteers, some with medical conditions such as irritable bowel syndrome or pain syndromes, showed improved energy and mood levels, as well as a decrease in depressive and anxiety symptoms (Horowitz, 2015).

Depression

Studies have been conducted for over fifty years on the effects of fasting on mood disorders. Recently, these studies have shifted to studying the effects of intermittent fasting on mood disorders and depression. These recent studies have found that participants had increased energy levels, as well as a reduction in anxiety and depression. One study found that intermittent fasting in men resulted in a decrease in body weight, body fat, and depression, thus giving them a perceived increase in their quality of life. Findings have indicated that intermittent fasting produces antidepressant-like effects. This has led to the theory that intermittent fasting could help with bipolar disorder, as it has been seen to reduce both the manic and depressive phases of this disorder (Horowitz, 2015).

Sleep

Even our sleeping bodies can benefit from fasting. Short term fasting has been reported to help improve sleep. It can lessen the amount of time we awake during the night, the amount of time we spend in REM sleep, and the amount of leg movements we experience. Eating in the evening can often cause problems with sleep, because your body is digesting when it should be in repair mode. This is one thing to think about if you are considering the Warrior Diet, as that fasting regimen requires eating during a short period of time in the evening (Breus, 2019).

No matter which fasting diet you choose, being in tune with your body is the best way to ensure a good night's sleep. Listen to your body, if you have a hard time sleeping and you eat in the evening, then adjust your eating window. That is one of the great things about intermittent fasting; as long as you stay inside that eating window, you will get results. You may need to have your first meal earlier in the day so that your last meal is further away from your bedtime. If possible, you may need to shift your sleep times and wake times, so that they better align with the fasting diet you are following. No matter what your eating window or sleeping time is, be sure to stay hydrated. Dehydration can cause you to wake at night. During non-fasting days, make sure you are still eating healthy foods. If you are eating foods with a lot of sugar or caffeine, it will negatively affect your sleep (Breus, 2019).

Skin

There are plenty of reports of fasting clearing up acne and improving the overall condition of participants' skin. While there has been no research on this directly, it makes sense that this would be the case. Fasting affects your blood glucose levels, and when your blood glucose levels are too high, your skin becomes dry and can cause collagen damage. Collagen is a protein that gives our skin its elasticity and fullness. Collagen also needs sugar, but when blood sugar is too high, glycation happens. This means that your collagen has taken in the wrong kind of sugar. Over time, these bad sugars can make your skin stiffen and appear aged (Fast Fix: Does, n.d.).

LONG TERM BENEFITS

While most people are looking for short term results, science has shown that there are many long term benefits associated with fasting, as well. All of the short term benefits listing above cause changes in our body's functioning and composition. These short term benefits, if maintained, will lead to long term benefits for our bodies. This will help us live longer, healthier, more active and disease free, thus more enjoyable, lives.

Metabolic Syndrome

Metabolic syndrome results in the accumulation of several conditions a person may have, such as, increased blood sugar, high blood pressure, high cholesterol or triglyceride levels, and excess fat around your middle section. These conditions increase your chances of stroke, heart attack, and type 2 diabetes. Having one of these conditions does not mean you have metabolic syndrome, but the more of these conditions you have, the higher your chances of developing type 2 diabetes or heart disease (Metabolic Syndrome - Symptoms, 2019).

Metabolic Syndrome is linked to being overweight and inactive. It is also linked to insulin resistance. When you are insulin resistant, your cells do not react how they should to insulin and it is hard for glucose to enter your cells. As a result, your blood sugar levels rise and your body continues to produce insulin to deal with the rising blood sugar levels. We have already looked at the effect fasting has on insulin; it helps stabilize both blood sugar and insulin levels (Metabolic Syndrome - Symptoms, 2019).

Chronic Inflammation

Chronic inflammation refers to your body's means of healing itself. It is how your body fights off such things as infections, injuries or toxins. When something damages your cells your body sends a message to your immune system, which in turn releases antibodies, proteins, and increased blood flow to the damaged cells. This process can last from a few days to a few weeks (Santos-Longhorn, 2018).

Chronic inflammation occurs when we remain in this state, an extended state of alertness. Over time, this can lead to damage to the cells of your organs and tissues. Acute inflammation can be easily identified by pain, redness, or swelling around the damaged cells. Chronic inflammation, however, is harder to identify, but does have some obvious symptoms. These symptoms, according to Santos-Longhurst include, "fatigue, fever, mouth sores, rashes, abdominal pain, and chest pain. These symptoms can range from mild to severe, and can last for several months or years (Healthline, 2018). Obesity is one of the main causes of chronic inflammation.

Researchers at Mount Sinai have found that fasting reduces inflammation and chronic inflammation without affecting the immune system's response to acute infections. Intermittent fasting reduces the release of monocytes (pro-inflammatory cells) into the blood. These monocytes are highly inflammatory immune cells that can cause serious damage. We have already discussed how fasting can reduce inflammation in the body through increasing our levels of ghrelin, the hunger hormone which also has an anti- inflammatory effect on the body (Santos-Longhorn, 2018).

Hepatic Steatosis

Intermittent fasting can help people prone to hepatic steatosis, or fatty liver disease. Fatty liver disease occurs when excess fat cells accumulate in the liver. While most people have no symptoms or complications, it can lead to liver disease. There are three stages in the development of fatty liver disease to liver disease. The first stage is called steato-hepatitis. Your liver will become swollen, in turn damaging the tissue. Then you enter a process called fibrosis, where scar tissue will form on the damaged tissue. The final stage, cirrhosis of the liver, occurs when the scar tissue replaces the healthy tissue. This scar tissue can eventually block liver function entirely. This can eventually lead to liver failure and liver cancer. You are more likely to develop hepatic steatosis if you have any of the following conditions - obesity, type 2 diabetes, insulin resistance, or metabolic syndrome (Fatty Liver Disease, 2020).

From what you have learned so far, each and every one of the conditions that can predispose you to fatty liver disease can be prevented or reduced through intermittent fasting. Also, as shown in the science behind intermittent fasting, when the body fasts and enters ketosis, the liver releases fatty acids. This process plus the weight loss (obesity is a major contributor to fatty liver disease) that results from ketosis, can help protect against this disease.

Heart Disease

Heart disease has many contributing factors, which probably explains why it is the leading cause of death around the world. One of the causes of heart disease is cholesterol levels.

Studies have shown that fasting can decrease levels of bad cholesterol (LDL) and blood triglycerides. Triglycerides are fats stored in your blood; a buildup of these can lead to heart disease. Fasting can also decrease blood pressure. The higher your blood pressure, the harder your heart has to work to pump blood throughout your body. Decreasing your blood pressure means your heart doesn't have to work so hard. As discussed earlier, fasting can help prevent and control diabetes, which is also a major contributor to heart disease (Fung, 2016).

These are some findings for studies conducted in 2017. Research was conducted on patients evaluated for heart disease in Utah and other Rocky Mountain states. The group included hundreds of Mormons, who typically fast one Sunday a month for up to 24 hours. These were the results of those studies, as reported by The American Heart Association News:

- In the first study they looked at how fasting affects life shape. They studied about 2000 people who had experienced cardiac catheterization for approximately 4.4 years. Three hundred eighty-nine of these participants had been routine fasters for at least the past five years. Researchers found that routine fasters had a 45% lower mortality rate than non-fasters.

- A second study used the same patient data, and after making the necessary adjustments, showed that routine fasters had 71 percent lower rate of developing heart failure than no-fasters.

Of course, a major consideration in the research group in this study is that they were mostly all members of the Church of Jesus Christ of Latter Day Saints and thus not necessarily eating the same foods or living the same lifestyle of the average American (Marshall, n.d.).

Degenerative Brain Disorders

There have been recent studies that have shown that fasting can have a positive effect on our brains, thus preventing some neurodegenerative disorders. While most these studies have been conducted on mice and not humans the results are positive, showing improved brain structure and brain function. These results have led researchers to be hopeful that fasting can help with disorders such as Parkinson's and Alzheimer's. This promising affect can be seen through the role of autophagy (Fung, 2016).

As we discussed earlier, fasting promotes autophagy, the process whereby damaged cell parts are replaced by new components. This can be directly related to degenerative brain disorders. When your body can't rebuild or get rid of damaged cells, they build up and can cause brain disorders like Alzheimer's. One of the causes of Alzheimer's is the build up of abnormal proteins that gum up the brain system. So, it makes sense that increased autophagy would replace these abnormal proteins and prevent the development of Alzheimer's (Fung, 2016c).

Psychological Disorders

One study showed improved psychological well-being, with participants decreased depression and binge eating, as well as a healthier self image. While studies have yet to be conducted on humans, rats and animals on IF have shown a longer lifespan than those on a non-fasting diet.

Cancer

There has only been one study conducted on the effects of intermittent fasting on breast cancer recurrence and the results were promising. Results of this study indicated that if the fasting period was more than 13 hours and occurring during your sleeping hours, it could decrease the chances of breast cancer recurrence in women. Our bodies are used to eating during the day time and fasting at night. Eating at irregular times can misalign our circadian rhythms. This disruption in our circadian rhythms has been linked to many forms of cancer (Rethink Breast Cancer, 2021).

Studies have also indicated that there could be benefits of fasting for those who are taking treatments for cancer. Some actually indicated that fasting was just as effective as chemo-therapy in slowing tumor growth. No such research, however, has been conducted on humans. Some cancer patients undergoing chemotherapy have practiced intermittent fasting while in treatment and stated that it did lessen the adverse side effects of chemo (Rethink Breast Cancer, 2021).

4

INTERMITTENT FASTING

There are many different options when choosing intermittent fasting. There is no right or wrong, better or best. It is up to personal preference. Whichever one fits into your life and your preferences is the one you will have the most success with.

The science supporting intermittent fasting stresses the importance of the changes that occur inside your body when you switch from eating to fasting. Intermittent fasting appears to have psychological benefits because cells undergo mild stress when we fast. Our body is preprogrammed to deal with these stressors, so it adapts. As long as we give the body time to adapt and deal with these stressors, this would be our non-fasting days, the body gets stronger. This continues every time we fast, thus improving our ability to cope, and perhaps resists some diseases (Collier, 2013).

When we eat, we are consuming three different types of macronutrients- carbohydrates, proteins and fats. Carbohydrates are the easiest macronutrient to breakdown into glucose, which is why we often see the restriction of carbs in other diet plans. We often take in more calories than we need at the time, so the body stores excess glucose in the liver and muscles. When we fast, the brain sends a message to the liver telling it to break down the glucose it has stored in the body. When the liver does this, it is said the body is entering a state of ketosis. When in ketosis, the body releases a fatty acid called ketones into the blood. These ketones have been shown to positively affect memory and learning, as well as slow certain brain diseases (Richter, 2020).

Also of importance here, as already discussed under general fasting, is that when your body is fasting, it has to use stored fat as an energy source. Most people store their fat in pockets around their midsection. This is particularly unhealthy because this is where your vital organs are located. When you fast, you are breaking down this fat stored around your organs, thus losing harmful body fat, not simply water weight or muscle mass.

TIME RESTRICTED FASTING

Timed fasting and intermittent fasting is often lumped into the same category but they are quite different. With time restricted fasting, all of your eating is within a particular time frame. Timed fasting can be anywhere from sixteen hours to three months or more! Intermittent fasting, on the other hand, can take on several forms, such as alternate day fasting or the 5:2 method. These will be discussed later.

16:8 or the Lean Gains Protocol

This is the most common type, fast for 16 hours, then eat all meals within an eight hour time period. Generally, you would eat your first meal at 11 am and your last meal at 7 pm. Most people using this fasting method usually skip breakfast and just eat two main meals. You do not have to be limited to two meals. However, if you prefer three, just eat three smaller ones, spaced out during an eight hour window Muszalski, 2019).

In addition to the health benefits and long term mental benefits already discussed, this particular method is promoted as the best to keep and build muscle mass. Studies have shown that performance is not negatively affected on this plan, and many actually report having more energy and mental clarity. It saves time, as you only prepare two meals a day as opposed to three and it's flexible as you can have your eating window any time of the day (Muszalski, 2019).

20:4 or the Warrior Diet

Inspired by ancient warriors, who ate all their meals in a four hour period in the evening. This is a very extreme form of timed intermittent fasting. During your 20 hour fast, if you eat anything it will just be a few pieces of raw fruit or vegetables. During the eating period, you would consume plenty of vegetables, proteins, healthy fats, and some carbohydrates. The 20:4 fasting diet is only recommended for those who have tried other intermittent fasting diets (Kubala, 2019).

The purpose of both of these fasts is the same, to lower insulin levels. Extended periods of low insulin will prevent the body from developing insulin resistance. Short periods of fasting can also reverse low levels of insulin resistance that may already be occurring in our bodies. A few small and reasonable snacks are allowed during the fasting hours. Many who try this diet experience a significant increase in energy during the day as well as an increase in the amount of fat lost per week (Fung, 2016b).

The Warrior Diet with its short window of eating, does not appear to be as sustainable as the 16:8 timed fast. There are also concerns about the amount of fiber you can consume in such a short period, as it's well known a lack of fiber in our diet is directly linked to some cancers. Many participants found it hard to eat so close to bedtime. It has been reported that it negatively affected their sleep. Others complained that it interfered with their social lives, as when they would normally go out, would be during their eating window (Kubala, 2019).

24 Hour Fast

On this fasting option, many fast from lunch to lunch (meaning you would skip dinner and breakfast) or dinner to dinner (you skip breakfast and lunch). This diet is similar to the Warrior Diet, as you are technically not going 24 hours without eating, but there is more flexibility in when you can eat. You can drink water, coffee or tea (no additives) during your fasting time. You eat what you normally would eat on your non-fasting days. This fasting diet focuses on calorie reduction, not restriction of certain foods (Fung, 2016b).

This timed fasting has several advantages among the longer fasts. You are technically eating everyday, therefore you are free to take any medications that require you to take them with food. In our society, most people eat their dinner as the main meal of the day, sitting down with their families. For many, breakfast is a grab and go, and lunch is eaten sitting at a desk. This diet allows you to still have that sit down meal with your family and the skipped meals will not really affect your daily routine (Fung, 2016b).

For weight loss, this 24 hour fast is recommended three times a week, but some people find it easy to incorporate into their work schedules, so actually fast five days a week, while they are at work.

Beyond 24 Hours

There are greater benefits to fasting beyond 24 hours, but there are greater risks, as well. The biggest risk may be for those on medication. Many medications must be taken with food to decrease or alleviate their side effects. If you are a diabetic, you definitely should not try to fast beyond 24 hours without the supervision of your doctor. If you take insulin and do not eat, your insulin dosage needs to be regulated, if not you may become hypoglycemic, which can be very dangerous (Fung, 2016b).

A 36 hour fast means that you go one entire day without eating. For example, if you eat your last meal at dinner on day one, you will not eat breakfast, lunch or dinner the following day. You will not eat until breakfast on day three. The next option is a 42 hour fast, and so on, (the world record being 382 days!). Calories are not restricted during your eating times on these extended fasts, but participants often report that their appetites actually decrease. This is because as you break the insulin resistance cycle, insulin levels decrease. As insulin levels decrease, appetite is suppressed, but energy expended stays the same or goes up (Fung, 2016b).

EXTENDED FASTING

The most obvious reason behind extended fasting is weight loss. During the first day of fasting, your body will use up the glucose in your liver and will then need to start breaking down the protein and fat stored in your body. While this may sound like what you want to happen, it can be dangerous. First, your body will turn to muscle mass, which we do not want broken down, as we need it, especially the muscle that is our heart! Then it will enter a state of ketosis, when it will finally start to break down our stored fat cells, and our weight loss will slow, but still occur at a rapid level. Staying in ketosis for a long time will result in a significant weight loss, but what happens when you start eating again? Many people simply go back to their old eating habits and they gain all the weight back again (Fung, 2016b).

History has shown that extended fasting can be dangerous. Heart failure can occur if potassium and magnesium levels in the body become depleted. You become more susceptible to infectious diseases because your body is not able to fight them off. Besides life threatening conditions, you may have to live with symptoms that are life altering at worst, irritating at best. Some of these are dizziness, lightheadedness, nausea, fainting, and chronic malnutrition.

Eat-Stop-Eat

This fasting method was first founded by Brad Pilon while he was doing research on fasting. It promotes fasting for 24 hours once or twice a week. For example, you would eat lunch on Monday at 12:00 PM, then you would fast until the following day, Tuesday 12:00 PM. At 12:00 PM that day you would eat your lunch, then you would eat dinner around 6:00 PM. You would then enter a 16:8 intermittent fasting method. So, you would fast from 6:00 PM Tuesday, until 10:00 AM the following day, Wednesday. On Wednesday, you would have an 8 hour eating window, starting with brunch at 10:00 AM, dinner at 6:00 PM. You can follow this same window the following day, Thursday, with brunch at 10:00 am and dinner at 6:00 PM. Then you can start another 24 hour fast at 6:00 PM on Thursday and fast until 6:00 PM on Friday. On this diet you are supposed to eat whatever you would normally eat on your non-fasting days. As such, there is no available meal plan for this method of fasting. Just follow the general advice on breaking your fast and introduce easily digestible, healthy food into your body first (Pilon, 2018).

Skipping Meals

Skipping meals and intermittent fasting is not the same thing. Forgetting to eat, being too busy to eat, or punishing yourself for gaining weight is not the same as practicing mindful eating. Skipping meals with no routine of plan can make you tired, sluggish and dizzy. When people just randomly skip meals, they tend to overeat at the next meal. If your meals are unpredictable, then your body will not know when to expect food again and it will slow your metabolism down, the opposite of what you need to lose weight. With intermittent fasting, your body becomes accustomed to the eating schedule and it knows food is coming so it will use stored fat until that food arrives (Shulman, 2019).

Irregularly skipping meals, if done on purpose and with a plan, can be a method of intermittent fasting. If you want to try intermittent fasting but you are not sure about your ability to persevere, or if you have an unpredictable schedule, this may be the diet for you. While a set fasting routine will give you the best results, fasting occasionally will still give you some benefits. This is a great way to introduce your body to intermittent fasting.

5:2 Diet

This diet allows you to eat what you want for five days and fast for two. The only restrictions on this diet is that participants consume their normal calories on the five eating days, and they eat 25% of their normal calorie intake on their fast days (500 calories for women, 700 calories for men). This diet is popular with first time dieters because it is easy to follow. The key to success in this diet seems to be knowing when to pick your two fast days. It is important to note that they do not have to be two consecutive days. So, you can fast on Monday, eat regularly on Tuesday, Wednesday, fast on Thursday, eat regularly Friday, Saturday, and Sunday. You could fast two days in a row. You can change it up if you wish (Bjarnadottir & Kubala, 2020).

Alternate Day Fasting (ADF)

On this diet, you fast every second day and eat what you want every other day. On fasting days, you drink as much calorie free beverages as you want, such as black unsweetened coffee, tea, and water. If you are following an altered fasting diet, you can eat approximately 500 calories a day. This alternate fasting day, however, does not seem to have the same results on weight loss as a complete fast would, but it does appear to be more sustainable. On your non-fasting days, you can eat what you want, but don't eat more than you normally would. In other words do not binge eat (Bjar-nadottir & Kubala, 2020).

Alternate Day Fasting, while effective in weight loss, has not been proven to be any more effective than reducing the daily amount of calories you consume. Nor has it been proven to be any better at reducing belly fat, inflammatory markers or maintaining muscle mass. It is also recommended that you partake in endurance exercise while ADF, as it will increase your amount of weight loss (Bjarnadottir & Kubala, 2020).

There are mixed results regarding hunger while on fasting days. Some studies say hunger levels decreased, while others say they stayed at the same level throughout. According to Bjarnadottir and Kubals, while ADF may be similar to daily calorie reduction when it comes to weight loss, one study showed increased levels of brain derived neurotrophic factor (BDNF) after 24 weeks of followup. BDNF influences energy levels and body weight maintenance. Researches stated that ADF may result in improved weight loss mainte-nance (Healthline, 2020).

The alternate version of this diet is known as the every-other-day fasting method and was established by Dr. Krista Varady, an assistant professor at University of Illinois. She found that women should eat 500-600 calories a day when they fast and men 700-900 calories on days they fast. On non-fasting days, you can eat anything you want and as much as you want (Bjarnadottir & Kubala, 2020).

SUCCESSFUL FASTING

As with any change we try to make to our lifestyle, there will be struggles to adapt, especially in the early stages. Knowledge is the key to success in many aspects of our life. In this section of "The Fasting Fact," we will look at some tips and products that will help you be successful while fasting. Be sure to read to the end of "The Fasting Facts" for some common myths about dieting; it may change your mind if you are still holding back from taking the plunge.

EATING WHILE INTERMITTENT FASTING

There are things that you can eat on your fast days, but just as important are the foods you eat on your non-fasting days. It is important that you do not view these days as binge days, but instead eat healthy until you are satisfied.

Many experts say that as long as you keep your caloric intake below 50 grams a day, your body will stay in ketosis. You can drink as much plain or carbonated water as you want, as well as coffee or tea, without milk or sugar (you can add a little milk or fat). Putting one or two teaspoons of apple cider vinegar in a glass of water can prevent food cravings for some people. Healthy fats, such as coconut oil, ghee or butter in your coffee or tea can help curb your hunger, as well. Bone broth can help you replace certain electrolytes lost during fasting and help you feel stated. While the healthy fats and bone broth will technically break your fast, if you keep the amounts small, it will not affect your body's ketosis (Panoff, 2019).

For people who already have a diet low in vitamins and minerals, while highly unlikely, could experience a deficiency in nutrients while fasting. These are some supplements that you should avoid while fasting. Gummy multivitamins, as these contain small amounts of sugar, protein and fat. Branched-chain amino acids, because these can trigger an insulin response that goes against autophagy. Protein powders, since these contain calories and can send a message to your body that you are not fasting. Finally, supplements that contain maltodextrin, pectin, sugar cane or fruit juice, all of which contains sugar and calories. All of these will technically break your fast (Panoff, 2019).

Supplements that are less likely to break your fast include multivitamins that do not contain sugar or fillers and few to no calories, Fish or algae oil in small doses, individual micronutrients, potassium, vitamins B and D. Creatine and pure collagen, as well as probiotics and prebiotics all are calorie free and will not interfere with insulin or ketosis (Panoff, 2019).

EXERCISING WHILE INTERMITTENT FASTING

Your exercise routine should be considered before you start intermittent fasting, as well. You don't want to give up one healthy activity for the sake of another. You need to think about when you normally work out. Which time frame would it best fall into? Pre- fasting, during your fasting window, or during your eating window? Ask yourself, do I prefer to work out shortly after I eat, right before I eat, or somewhere in the middle? That is the great thing about the 16:8 method, it gives you the flexibility to move your fasting period around your exercise routine if you can't move your exercise routine around your fasting window (Bubnis, 2020).

Moderate to High Intensity Exercise

What you eat is important to your exercise routine as well. The macronutrients you take in before your fasting workout will determine the effectiveness of your workout. Strength workouts will require more carbs before, while low intensity or cardio workouts will require fewer carbs. What you eat after your workout is as important as what you eat before. If you are performing weightlifting exercises, it is important to have protein to repair muscle after a workout (Lindberg, 2020).

Tips for Doing Moderate to High Intensity Exercise

You can continue to exercise while fasting. The question lays more in the sustainability of the two combined, more so than one over the other. If your goal is to lose body fat and maintain a physically active lifestyle, Lindberg (2020) recommends you follow these suggestions:

- Eat a meal close to any high to moderate intensity workout. This will give your body the necessary fuel it needs, without breaking down muscle or causing you to 'hit a wall' during your workout.

- Drink water. Water does not break your fast and you need it during exercise even more.
- Coconut water is a great way to replenish your electrolytes without consuming many calories. Stay away from popular sports drinks as they are high in sugar.
- Listen to your body. If you get dizzy or lightheaded, stop and take a break.
- If you are doing a 24 hour fast, consider walking, pilates, or restorative yoga instead of your current exercise routine.

Intensive exercise is not recommended during your fasting period, however. This may cause your body to break down muscle mass and access to protein based food directly after intense exercise is necessary to repair muscle breakdown. So, if you plan on doing activities that require a high amount of strength or speed, or those that continue for an extensive period of time, you need a readily available energy source. Keep these activities for your non-fasting days (Lindberg, 2020).

Cardiovascular Exercise

It has been shown that performing cardio while fasting can help you burn more fat. Not having excess calories to use for fuel during your workout means the body has to use stored glucose and fat to get the energy it needs. Some studies show that if you workout first thing in the morning after a 8-10 hour fast, you can burn up to 20 % more fat. This would certainly support hopping on your treadmill or elliptical during your fasting times (Lindberg, 2020).

The best way to know what exercise you can handle while intermittent fasting is to try it. Your body will tell you what you can handle and what you cannot. Doing cardio while fasting requires you to be in excellent physical health, which is not necessarily determined by your weight. If you experience any dizziness from sudden drops in blood pressure or blood sugars while exercising, it can be very dangerous (Lindberg, 2020).

Tips for Doing Cardio While Fasting

If you want to try cardio exercises while fasting the following, according to Lindberg (2020) will help you success:

- Keep it to 60 minutes or less.
- Workouts should be moderate to low intensity.
- Don't forget to hydrate. Fasting cardio includes drinking water.
- Remember that your lifestyle and overall nutrition will be a bigger determinant to your weight loss than exercising will.

Above all, listen to your body. If you do not feel well, you are dizzy, get a headache, or you feel nauseous during or directly after performing cardio during fasting, then it is not for you.

HOW TO BREAK YOUR FAST EFFECTIVELY

When you start to introduce food back into your diet, be sure to do it slowly, in small portions of foods that can be easily digested. Avoid foods that are high in sugar, fat, and fiber. Foods that normally are viewed as 'good' foods can be hard on your body and cause a lot of discomfort when digested, such as nuts and raw fruits and vegetables, due to their high fiber content. These are some of the foods that would be easily introduced into your diet:

- Smoothies, as they contain less fiber than raw produce.
- Dried fruit, like dates, apricots, and raisins
- Soups, made with legumes or pasta. Do not eat soups with heavy creams and raw vegetables.
- Well cooked starchy vegetables, such as potatoes.
- Fermented foods, such as unsweetened yogurt and kefir.
- Healthy fats, such as eggs and avocados (Panoff, 2019).

Once you are able to eat these with no discomfort add other healthy foods such as beans, whole grains, meat, and fish. As important as what you eat, is how much you eat. Do not overeat during your non-fasting period. If you binge eat, especially on high sugar and processed carbohydrates, you risk reversing all the good done during your fast (Panoff, 2019).

APPS TO HELP YOU ON YOUR JOURNEY

How often do we leave the house without our phones? We use apps for work, social media, news feeds, so why not to help us on our journey to a healthier life? These are a few of the recommended apps, from Women's Health (Bradley & Miller 2121) you can download on your phone, so that you can get the assistance and encouragement you may need anywhere you go.

- **Window**: This app has a variety of tools to make intermittent fasting easy for you. Schedule your eating window, receive notification when it opens and closes, sync with apple health, and it gives you healthy suggestions. There is also a premium version, which you pay for. This version lets you choose your plan, upload photos, track your weight, and attach daily notes. Available for IOS and Android.

- **Infasting:** Just some of the features of Infasting include a journal, calendar to track your body changes, daily logs, and reminders. Only available for IOS.

- **Fastic:** Will keep you on track with your eating. Over 400 recipe ideas, with healthy, filling ingredients. It also gives you information on IF, has a step counter, and allows you to connect with other intermittent fasters. IOS and Android versions available.

- **Zero:** Can be customized to your fasting plan. You can choose from several preprogrammed fasting windows or program your own fasting up to one week. Easy to use and can help you analyze your fasting habits. Available for IOS and Android.

- **Fastient:** One of the most comprehensive tracking apps. It allows you to track all your food intake and track your progress. Easy to use, so that you can journal, follow your data in graphs, view your information on a mobile device or your desktop. You can change your goals or change your method of intermittent fasting. Compatible for IOS or Android.

WOMEN VS MEN

Losing weight is not easy for anyone, man or woman. We often see couples go on diets together and the weight drops off of the husband faster than the wife. Does the husband have more willpower? Is the wife giving in and cheating behind his back? As we all know, life is not fair. Especially a life where you are struggling to control your weight. Yes, men and women do lose weight differently.

Men do lose weight faster than women; it's simply physiology. Men have a higher metabolism and produce more lean muscle mass than women. Men also carry their weight around their midsection, which is more dangerous, but is a better place to store it when it comes to weight loss. When men burn this visceral fat, it boosts their metabolism, making them burn even more fat. Women, on the other hand, store their excess fat as subcutaneous fat, around their hips and thighs. Unfortunately, this fat does not affect metabolic rate. So, as one can see, men and women's bodies are different and that affects how they lose weight. That is not to say that women cannot benefit from intermittent fasting (Orlando, 2020).

To understand how men and women's bodies respond to food, we can look at cultural roles over time, as well. Back in "hunter and gatherer" society, humans fasted because they had to, not because they chose to. There were periods of plenty and periods of scarcity. Men, with their larger physical size and strength, responded to this scarcity with a burst in their metabolic rate. Then, they had the necessary energy to go out and hunt for the entire clan. Their bodies responded to hunger by creating energy so that they could go out and get more food to satisfy that hunger (Orlando, 2020). Research shows that this genetic predisposition still exists today. A man's metabolic rate can increase up to 14% on a 12-14 hour fast. Men also get the benefit of testosterone utilization increasing by 10-200%, and a 100-200% improvement in HGH.

Women's bodies, however, responded differently to periods of scarcity by slowing down levels of metabolism. The body does this to conserve energy and store fat in order to survive a potential extended period without food. What this means is that today, intermittent fasting may not have the same results for women as it does for men (Intermittent Fasting: Women, n.d.).

While intermittent fasting can be beneficial for both men and women, intermittent fasting may be harder on women than men. This is due to the hormones involved. Women have higher levels of a protein called kisspeptin, which causes greater sensitivity to fasting. It has also been suggested that due to reproductive hormones, women may have greater difficulty controlling hunger while fasting (English, 2019).

While men's nervous systems appear to become less agitated during fasting, women's appear to become more agitated. Another study showed that women's levels of good cholesterol (HDL) increased more with intermittent fasting, than it did in men. Also, women's triglycerides levels lowered at a greater level than men, meaning women may benefit more from IF when it comes to risk of heart disease and stroke (intermittent Fasting: Women, n.d.).

Intermittent fasting has been shown to impact the hunger hormones, leptin and ghrelin. Leptin is made by fat cells and helps decrease your hunger. Ghrelin, however, increases your appetite. Levels of leptin are actually lowered when you are thin and are higher when you are fat. Many people who are obese, seem to have built up a resistance to leptin. Normally, ghrelin levels go up before you eat, signaling your brain that you are hungry. Once you eat, ghrelin levels go down and stay level for about three hours after you eat. Studies have shown that shorter fasting periods, under 24 hours, will result in having longer periods of low amounts of ghrelin after you eat. So, in short, fasting can help lessen your hunger and appetite, thus help you lose weight. Some studies have shown that women may benefit more for a constant decrease in calorie intake, than a complete fasting period (Intermittent Fasting: Women, n.d.).

Modified Approach to Fasting for Women

One study showed blood sugar control worsened for women over a three week period but got better for men. Many women noted changes to their menstrual cycles. When calorie intake is low, the hypothalamus is affected. This can result in the disruption of two reproductive hormones, which control the ovaries. The result is irregular periods, infertility and poor bone health. For these reasons, women should consider shorter fasting periods or fewer fasting days. That is not to say women should not partake in intermittent fasting (Intermittent Fasting: Women, n.d.).

There are benefits for women who intermittently fast, especially if you are not of child baring years. Not only can intermittent fasting shrink your waistline, it can help lower your chances of heart disease. Intermittent Fasting has been proven to lower blood pressure, LDL cholesterol and triglycerides.

BEST FASTING METHOD FOR BUILDING MUSCLE

The 16:8, or leangain, method is the best intermittent fasting for the athlete or anyone who wishes to build more muscle mass. This method actually began in the strength building community. Martin Berkhan, a Swedish powerlifter, went against the popular trend of the day, eating several small meals throughout the day, and promoted the 16 hour fasting period, followed by the 8 hour eating window. With his daily fasting, he was able to achieve 5.5% body fat. While we know fasting has been around for centuries, it was Berkhan in the 2000s who got the world's attention by showing us that fasting could also improve our body composition and strength (Graeme, 2019).

Because the leangain method does not require long periods of fasting, you can continue to workout as you normally would. We know that fasting is one way to deal with insulin sensitivity, but it is also believed to improve the way our body absorbs nutrients and our body's composition. Exercising during fasting has been shown to burn fat faster than exercising when you are not fasting. Fasting appears to increase adrenaline, which increases fat oxidation. Some studies have shown that fasting may help preserve muscle mass while fasting. It is believed that weight training while fasting can stimulate muscle gain and human growth hormone, which retains muscle (Graeme, 2019).

WORKING OUT WHILE ON LEANGAIN FASTING METHOD

The Leangain workout plan is simple, low volume, and focuses on powerlifting movements. According to barbend.com, you work out three days a week, and each day focuses on a different area of your body:

- Back day: deadlift, overhead pass, weighted chin ups, rows, body weight chin ups.
- Chest day: bench press, incline dumbbell press, bicep curls, tricep extensions.
- Leg day: squat, hamstring curl, leg extension, cable crunch, calf raises.

Berkhan also applies a reverse pyramid method to his training. Three warm up sets of 40, 60, and 80% of working weight. Followed by a heavy working set (with 3-5 reps for the deadlift and 6-10 reps for all other exercises). The weight is then decreased by 10%, and you take a rest for 3-5 minutes, and complete a second set with one more rep. Then you repeat this one more time (Graeme, 2019).

If you are working out during your eating window, he suggests you have a small meal an hour or two prior to working out. If working out during your fasting window, you should take amino acid supplements. According to

Graeme, (2019) these are the supplements recommended if working out while fasting on the leangain method:

- Essential Amino Acids: The building blocks of protein, they may improve performance and maintain muscle mass.
- Fish oil: Can help with muscle growth, as well as inflammation and immunity.
- Creatine: Improves muscle size and power output.
- Calcium: Good for bone health, may increase fat secretion and boost testosterone.
- Vitamin D: May help with athletic performance, immunity, bone health and boost testosterone.
- Glucosamine: Reduces joint pain.

THE FASTING PROCESS ITSELF

Now that you have educated yourself on intermittent fasting and decided to give it a shot, there are still a few steps you should take. The following is a combined list of all the advice from different experts in the field. Do the following to ensure that you get through the tough stage of your body adapting to a new eating schedule, once you do, it's smooth sailing.

BE HONEST WITH YOURSELF

Intermittent fasting has a variety of proven benefits for your body and mind, but it is not for everyone. Consider your own personal level of self-discipline and your relationship with food. Consider your level of exercise, your lifestyle, and anything else about your current situation that would make fasting difficult for you. Give it a try and if you fail, be honest as to why. Assess the situation and why you went wrong. Then try again.

WATCH YOUR BODY'S RESPONSE

Your body speaks volumes, especially to change. The beginning phase of intermittent fasting will give you the best information as to how to be successful. This first stage will be the hardest, as your body is adjusting to a new eating schedule, so pay attention to how you feel. Some discomfort will occur during the first three to four weeks, but any longer than that you need to see a doctor.

DO NOT EXPECT CONSISTENT WEIGHT LOSS RIGHT AWAY

Your body is going to experience fluctuations in hormone levels. With this fluctuation, your body will become a little confused in what to do with calories. Sometimes they will hold on to every calorie it has and other times you will lose weight. So, you will see an up and down situation when you step on the scales.

WATER

Drink a lot of water. Start this before you even begin to fast to get your body used to it. Drink at least a gallon of water a day. Not only is water beneficial to your health, but it will help you feel full while on your fast.

CAFFEINE

Research has shown that black coffee can suppress your appetite and it will not interfere with your fast, but only if your coffee has no sugar, artificial sweeteners or cream. This does not apply to coffee beverages, even if they say zero calories, they will still have additives that will break your fast and may be harmful to your health.

KEEP YOURSELF BUSY

Keeping busy will keep your mind off the fact that you are fasting. We want what we cannot have! If you are thinking about food, especially towards the end of your fasting period, you are going to crave it. If your mind is occupied with other duties, you will not think about food, and therefore not be tempted to break your fast.

START YOU FAST CORRECTLY

Once you have your last meal, your fasting begins. Brush your teeth to get the feel and taste of food out of your mind. Then occupy your mind. Schedule your daily chores and work routines around your fasting schedule. After you go through the fasting schedule several times, this will become second nature to you and you won't have to give it a thought.

INDIVIDUALIZE IT

One of the best things about intermittent fasting is it can work around any type of schedule. We all have one meal of the day that we "just can't miss", so don't! If you follow the 16:8 method or even the 20:4 method, it's the length of the eating window that matters, not the time of the day it occurs. Experiment until you find that window of time that works best for you.

SLOW AND STEADY

If you are finding it hard to skip a meal, try delaying it an hour at a time until it becomes the next meal. If you normally eat your breakfast at 7:00 AM and you simply can't go without, try eating it at 8:00 AM. Do this for a week. The next week, move it to 9:00 AM, the next week 10:00 AM. If you do this consistently, it will be 12:00 PM and lunch time! If you cannot go that long, move your lunch back as well, and eat a combined meal of brunch. This slow steady approach will be much easier on your body as well.

CHOOSE YOUR FRIENDS CAREFULLY

Sometimes your friends can make or break your diet. Although you may know of all the benefits of intermittent fasting, many people do not. Some people will be negative no matter what you try. While friends can be a great support system, they can also be very judgmental. Intermittent fasting is personalized to your schedule, so no one else should matter. Just as your weight loss is for you and no one else.

KICK YOUR DAY OFF WITH WATER

We already discussed the importance of water, but it cannot be stressed enough. Many times when you think you are hungry, you are actually thirsty. If you do not respond to these signals for water, your body will then send out hunger signals to get your attention. Remember, much of the water we get comes from the food we consume. If you are fasting, you need to make up for that missed water. So, start your day by drinking water as soon as you wake up. Drinking at least a half a liter or water upon waking refreshes your body and makes you feel full. Continue to drink water throughout the day, stopping a few hours before you go to sleep.

DO NOT OVEREXTEND YOURSELF

Even if you think fasting is not doing any harm to your body and you are feeling fine, never fast for more than two days straight. We are all different and our bodies all react differently at different times. Your body should undergo some changes when you first begin intermittent fasting, it just may take a little longer than most. Start with lower fast periods of 12, 14, then 16, or more. Try each interval a week at a time to allow your body to adjust. Intermittent fasting is not about seeing how long you can go without eating, it is simply giving your body a break from eating.

DO NOT DEPRIVE YOURSELF

While intermittent fasting does promote healthy eating when non-fasting, it is okay to treat yourself. If you want to eat that piece of cake, do it. Just remember what is needed to burn it back off. Perhaps most importantly, do not let that piece of cake knock you off track. Take it for what it is and move on. Even of more importance may be social contacts.

Do not let the fact that you are fasting force you to go without your social support system. We can not stress enough the flexibility of intermittent fasting. If you know you have a social engagement of celebration coming up, adjust your fasting window. Do not make a habit of this however, or you may end up with more eating windows, than fasting!

PROTEIN

Good quality protein is a very important part of your meals when you are intermittent fasting. Protein helps you stay full longer by reducing your level of ghrelin, the hunger hormone, and increasing your levels of peptide YY, the hormone that makes you feel satisfied. High quality steak and chicken will take hours for your body to digest, therefore making you feel full a lot longer than other foods. Protein is also critical for making your muscles stay strong and lean, which we want as we lose weight. So, if after several days, you are still feeling hungry during your fasting period, add some good quality protein to your next meal (Rios, 2017).

TAKE A BREAK

If you normally work out, you may need to take a break from strenuous exercise the first few times you fast. Remember, your body is no longer getting a direct, easily converted source of energy. It is working to create its own energy, that is less energy available for your activities. It is okay to take a long walk or to practice some yoga but strenuous activity is not recommended. After your body adjusts, you can work yourself up to your old routines.

BCAAS

Branched chain amino acids (BCAAs) can be good for those who want to continue to strength train during intermittent fasting. BCAAs have been shown to prevent the consumption of lean muscle mass, as the body tries to produce its own energy, while stimulating additional fat loss. This supplement is not recommended for the average person on intermittent fasting, just those who do a lot of strength training (Rios, 2017).

CHOOSE YOUR MEALS WISELY

While intermittent fasting does not require you to count calories, as most diets do, you still need to look at the quality of food you consume. You cannot use the excuse that you just skipped meals to load up on calories when you do eat, that will defeat the whole purpose! If you eat unhealthy food on your non-fasting days, you will reverse the good done in your body during your fasting days. Not only that, if you load up on high-sugar foods, it will make your fasting period harder, as your body will crave these foods.

BREAKING YOUR FAST

Breaking your fast properly is just as important as starting it properly. After fasting, it is especially important that you feed your body with the nutrients it needs. Eating healthy when you do eat, will also accelerate your weight loss. A smoothie is a great first meal after a fasting period, easily digestible and, if made with the right ingredients, nutrition packed. See the bonus section of this book for great smoothie recipes.

HEAD HUNGER VS BODY HUNGER

Listen to and get to know your body. Your mind often tells you that you are hungry when you are not. You may be thirsty, bored, upset, or simply stimulated because you smell food. When your body is hungry, you will feel differently; your stomach will 'growl' and let you know. Even then, that does not mean that you need to eat right away. You can go several days without food before your body experiences negative effects, so what harm will come from another hour or two?

CRAVINGS

Just because you crave something, doesn't mean you need it. Cravings make you think you are hungry when you really are not. What makes matters worse, is that we usually crave things we know are not healthy, so we try to satisfy that craving with something else. Of course, the craving doesn't go away, because we did not give ourselves what we truly wanted. If you must satisfy a craving, give yourself a little taste of that particular food, but only during your non-fasting period. Do not break your fast to give in to a craving. Do not let food control you.

RESPECT INTERMITTENT FASTING

Intermittent fasting is only as healthy as the person partici-pating makes it. If you have a history of eating disorders, do not try intermittent fasting. If you suffer from binge eating and purging, your mind can confuse it with intermittent fasting; it is not the same. Intermittent fasting is not extended fasting; you cannot go without eating for extended periods of time. Intermittent fasting is safe, and can be a part of a healthy lifestyle, if you practice it responsibly.

PLAN

It is evident that you have to plan ahead when intermittent fasting, you plan when you are going to eat and you need to have the best foods available to help you get the nutrients you need and the foods that will make you feel satisfied and keep you satisfied. Plus, foods to boost your metabolism is a huge plus if you are trying to lose weight. So, start by clearing low nutrient, high calorie junk food out of your house or at least out of your sight. Fill your kitchen with healthy, high nutrient foods. Plan your activities, especially social gatherings around your fasting window. If that can't be done, then more your fasting window.

HOW TO BOOST YOUR METABOLISM

While you will lose weight while intermittent fasting, specific foods can increase the amount of fat you lose. Make sure you have these items in your house when your fast ends. Already having these foods will prevent you from giving in to the temptation of eating low-density foods, restaurant food, or junk food.

PROTEIN RICH FOOD-YOUR BODY WILL NEED TO USE MORE ENERGY TO DIGEST THESE FOODS

- Eggs
- Nuts and Seeds - particularly almonds and walnuts
- Legumes - kidney beans, chickpeas, and lentils
- Fish - sardines, salmon, and other freshwater fish
- Meat - skinless chicken, lean beef, top sirloin, and beef tenderloin

These foods will fill you up faster, preventing you from overeating and keep you full longer. Protein rich foods also have what is known as a 'thermal' effect on your body. This thermal effect refers to the amount of energy your body uses to break down and absorb the nutrients in these foods. Your metabolism has to work faster when your body is digesting these protein rich foods. When your metabolism works faster, your body uses more energy, and you consume more calories, which means you will lose weight faster (Petre, 2016).

ESSENTIAL VITAMINS AND MINERALS

- Zinc
- Iron
- Selenium

These vitamins and minerals are necessary for the body to function properly. Diets lacking in zinc, iron, and selenium affect the thyroid gland. It reduces its ability to produce crucial hormones responsible for regulating your body's metabolism, causing it to slow down. These vitamins and minerals can best be found in nuts, seeds, legumes, meat, and seafood (Petre, 2016).

CHILI PEPPERS

Capsaicin is a chemical found in chili peppers that boosts the body's metabolism. This chemical will increase the calories and fat you burn while intermittent fasting. Add them to your food during your non-fasting period (Petre, 2016).

COFFEE

Already mentioned for its caffeine and the ability to suppress your appetite, it can also boost your metabolism. The caffeine in coffee is said to increase your metabolism by 11%. Studies have shown consuming three cups of black coffee a day can burn an additional 100 calories a day. Remember, no sugar or artificial sweeteners in your coffee, whether it is consumed on a fasting period or an eating period (Petre, 2016).

TEA

Tea has been known to have many health benefits; it provides antioxidants, reduces heart attacks and strokes, and can help protect your bones. Tea is also known to help with weight loss by boosting metabolism. Green and Oolong tea can be particularly beneficial and can burn up to 100 calories a day (Petre, 2016).

WHO SHOULD NOT FAST

As with any diet or lifestyle, certain people should not make changes without consulting their doctor or a designated medical professional. The same is true for any type of fasting. Fasting for a short period of time will not hurt anyone, especially if you stay properly hydrated. However, long term fasting, especially for those who have certain medical conditions or who are even predisposed to these conditions, can be dangerous. We know fasting can cause dips and spikes in blood sugar levels, so if you have diabetes or low blood sugar, do not fast. If you are pregnant or breastfeeding, you should not fast. Anyone with a chronic disease, the elderly, and children should not fast. This is because in these conditions and ages of growth and development, your body needs easy access to a fast and healthy supply of nutrients, vitamins, and minerals to aid in growth and rejuvenation. If you have an eating disorder, you should not fast. Long periods of fasting can lead to bingeing in those prone to eating disorders. Also, you may push yourself to fast too long, which can be dangerous.

CONCLUSION

While fasting is not for everyone, it may be the solution for you. With the short term benefits and the long term results of fasting, it is worth a try. You could lose weight, body fat, lower your blood pressure, and bad cholesterol levels. You may increase your levels of good cholesterol and stabilize your blood sugars. All of these benefits can lead to long term gain by lowering your chances of chronic disease and increasing longevity. Fasting only becomes dangerous if you fast for extended periods of time. So, respect the rules of fasting, follow the tips and plans given in "The Fasting Facts", and be healthy and happy!

SAMPLE 7 DAY INTERMITTENT FASTING MEAL PLAN

The following meal plan comes from www.WomensHealth-Mag.com. They are not listed by day, but by meal, so that you can mix and match to your liking. This meal plan would be for the most common type of intermittent fasting, 16:8; where you eat a late breakfast and dinner on your non-fasting days (Health, 2020).

BRUNCH RECIPES:

Scrambled Eggs with Sweet Potatoes

Total Time: 25 minutes

Serving Size: 1

Nutritional Facts:

calories: 571
carbs: 52g
fat: 20g
protein: 44g

Ingredients:

- 1 medium sweet potato, chopped
- ½ cup chopped onion
- 2 tsp chopped rosemary
- 4 large eggs
- 4 large egg whites
- 2 tbsp chopped chives
- Salt and pepper

Directions:

1. Preheat the oven to 425 degrees F.
2. Toss the sweet potato, onion, rosemary, and salt and pepper to taste in a bowl.
3. Spray a baking sheet with cooking spray.
4. Spread the potatoes out on the baking sheet.
5. Cook for about 20 minutes or until golden brown.
6. While the potatoes are roasting, beat the eggs, egg whites, and salt and pepper to taste in a medium sized bowl.
7. Spray a skillet with cooking spray.
8. A few minutes before the potatoes are done, scramble the eggs over medium heat.
9. Plate eggs and potatoes; sprinkle with chopped chives.

Greek Chickpea Waffles

Total Time: 30 minutes

Servings Size: 2

Nutritional Facts:

calories: 412
carbs: 24g
fat: 18 g
protein: 35g

Ingredients:

- ¾ cup chickpea flour
- ½ tsp baking soda
- ½ tsp salt
- ¾ cup Greek Yogurt, plain 2%
- 6 large eggs
- Tomatoes, cucumbers, scallion, olive oil, parsley, yogurt and lemon juice
- Salt and pepper

Instructions:

1. Preheat the oven to 200 degrees F. Place a wire rack over a baking sheet and place in the oven.
2. Heat the waffle iron.
3. Mix flour, baking soda, and salt in a large mixing bowl.
4. In a small mixing bowl, beat the eggs and whisk in yogurt.
5. Mix the wet ingredients into the dry until well blended.
6. Spray waffle iron with cooking spray.
7. Pour ¼ to ½ cup of batter into each section of the waffle iron.
8. Cook until golden brown, about 5 minutes.
9. Place cooked waffles in the oven to keep warm.
10. Repeat until all batter is used.
11. While waffles are cooking, chop tomatoes, cucumber, and scallion.
12. Toss vegetables with olive oil, parsley, yogurt and lemon juice, to your liking.
13. Top waffles with tomato mixture and enjoy.

PB&J Overnight Oats

Prep Time: 5 min (plus overnight in the refrigerator)

Serving Size: 1

Nutritional Facts:

> *calories: 455*
> *carbs 36g*
> *fat: 28g*
> *protein: 20g*

Ingredients:

- ¼ cup quick cooking rolled oats
- ½ cup 2% milk
- 3 tbsp creamy peanut butter
- ¼ cup mashed raspberries
- 3 tbsp whole raspberries

Instructions:

1. Combine oats, milk, peanut butter and mashed berries in a medium bowl. Stir until well blended.
2. Cover and place in the refrigerator overnight.
3. In the morning, remove the cover, top with whole raspberries and enjoy.

* * *

Turmeric Tofu Scramble

Total Time: 15 minutes

Serving Size: 1

Nutritional Facts:

calories: 431
carbs: 17g
fat: 33g
protein: 21g

Ingredients:

- 1 portobello mushroom
- 3-4 cherry tomatoes
- 1 tbsp olive oil (plus more for brushing)
- salt and pepper
- ¼ block (14 oz) firm tofu
- ¼ tsp ground turmeric
- pinch garlic powder
- ½ avocado, thinly sliced

Instructions:

1. Preheat the oven to 400 degrees F.
2. Place the mushroom and tomatoes on the baking sheet; brush with olive oil. Season with salt and pepper to taste.
3. Place in the oven and roast approximately 10 minutes or until tender.
4. While mushroom and tomatoes are roasting, mash the tofu, turmeric, garlic powder, and salt in a medium bowl.
5. In a large skillet, heat 1 tbsp of olive oil over medium heat. Add tofu and cook about 3 minutes, stirring occasionally, until firm.
6. Plate the tofu, serve with the roasted mushroom, tomato, and avocado slices.

* * *

Avocado Ricotta Power Toast

Total Time: 5 minutes

Serving Size: 1

Nutritional Facts:

> *calories: 288*
> *carbs: 9g*
> *fat: 17 g*
> *protein: 10g*

Ingredients:

- 1 slice whole grain bread
- ¼ ripe avocado, mashed
- 2 tbsp ricotta cheese
- pinch crushed red pepper flakes
- Pinch flaked sea salt

Instructions:

1. Toast the bread.
2. Top with avocado, cheese, red pepper, and salt.
3. Eat with scrambled or hard-boiled eggs, and a serving of yogurt or fruit.

Turkish Egg Breakfast

Total Time: 13 minutes

Serving Size: 2

Nutritional Facts:

calories: 469
carbs: 26g
fat: 29g
protein: 25g

Ingredients:

- 2 tbsp olive oil
- ¾ cup diced red bell pepper
- ¾ diced eggplant
- pinch of salt and pepper
- 5 large eggs, beaten
- ¼ tsp paprika
- chopped cilantro, to taste
- 2 dollops plain yogurt
- 1 whole wheat pita

Instructions:

1. Over medium heat, heat olive oil in a large skillet.
2. Add bell pepper, eggplant, and salt and pepper.
3. Cook until soft, approximately 7 minutes.
4. Stir in eggs, paprika, salt and pepper to taste.
5. Stirring often, cook until eggs are done.
6. Plate and top with chopped cilantro; serve with yogurt and pita.

* * *

Almond Apple Spice Muffins

Total Time: 15 minutes

Serving Size: 5

Nutrition Facts:

calories: 484
carbs: 16g
fat: 31g
protein: 40g

Ingredients:

- ½ stick butter
- 2 cups almond meal
- 4 scoops vanilla protein powder
- 4 large eggs
- 1 cup unsweetened applesauce
- 1 tbsp cinnamon
- 1 tsp allspice
- 1 tsp cloves
- 2 tsp baking powder

Instructions:

1. Preheat the oven to 350 degrees F.
2. In a microwave safe bowl, melt the butter in the microwave at 50% power, in 30 second increments.
3. In a large mixing bowl, mix the remaining ingredients with the melted butter.
4. Spray 2 muffin pans with cooking spray, or use paper liners.
5. Pour the batter into the muffin tins, until about ¾ full, making 10 muffins.
6. Place in the oven and bake for about 12 minutes or until a toothpick comes out clean.
7. Allow to cool before eating.

* * *

Dinner Recipes:

Turkey Tacos

Total Time: 25 minutes

Serving Size: 4

Nutritional Facts:

calories: 472
carbs: 30g
fat: 27g
protein: 28g

Ingredients:

- 2 tsp oil
- 1 small red onion, chopped
- 1 clove garlic, finely chopped
- 1 lb. ground turkey, extra-lean
- 1 tbsp sodium-free taco seasoning
- 8 whole-grain corn tortillas, warmed
- ¼ cup sour cream
- ½ cup shredded Mexican cheese
- 1 avocado, sliced
- Salsa
- 1 cup chopped lettuce

Instructions:

1. Using a large skillet on medium high heat, sauté onion in the oil about 5 minutes or until tender.
2. Add garlic and cook for another minute.
3. Add turkey and cook for about 5 minutes, or until nearly brown.
4. Add taco seasoning and 1 cup of water.
5. Simmer for about 7 minutes or until thickened.
6. Fill the tortillas with turkey. Top with the remaining ingredients.

* * *

Healthy Spaghetti Bolognese

Total Time: 1 hour 30 minutes

Serving Size: 4

Nutritional Facts:

calories: 450
carbs: 31g
fat: 23g
protein: 32g

Ingredients:

- 1 large spaghetti squash
- 3 tbsp olive oil
- ½ tsp garlic powder
- kosher salt and pepper
- 1 small onion, chopped
- 1 ¼ lb. ground turkey
- 4 cloves garlic, finely chopped
- 8 oz. small cremini mushrooms, sliced
- 3 cups fresh diced tomatoes
- 1 (8 0z) can low-sodium, no sugar-added tomato sauce
- fresh chopped basil

Instructions:

1. Preheat the oven to 400 degrees F.
2. Cut spaghetti squash in half lengthwise. Scoop out the seeds.
3. Rub each cut side with ½ tsp oil. Sprinkle it with garlic powder, and salt and pepper.
4. Place in a rimmed baking dish, cut side down.
5. Bake for 35 to 40 minutes or until tender.
6. Remove from the oven and let cool for 10 minutes.
7. In a large skillet, sauté onions, seasoned with salt and pepper, in 2 tbsp oil, over medium heat until tender.
8. Add turkey and cook for 6-7 minutes, until browned. Be sure to stir constantly to break up into small pieces.
9. Stir in garlic; cook for an additional minute.
10. Push the turkey to one side of the skillet and add the mushrooms to the other side. Cook and stir occasionally, until tender, about 5 minutes.
11. Mix mushrooms with the turkey. Add tomatoes and tomato sauce.
12. Simmer for 10 minutes.
13. While the sauce finishes, use a fork to shred the squash out of its shell. It will come out in long

strings, like spaghetti. Transfer to plate and top with Bolognese sauce. Sprinkle basil on the sauce, if desired.

* * *

Chicken with Fried Cauliflower Rice

Total time: 35 minutes

Serving Size: 4

Nutritional Facts:

calories: 427
carbs: 25g
fat: 16g
protein: 45g

Ingredients:

- 2 tbsp grapeseed oil
- 1 ¼ lb. boneless, skinless chicken breast
- 4 large eggs, beaten
- 2 red bell peppers, finely chopped
- 2 small carrots, finely chopped
- 1 onion, finely chopped
- 2 cloves garlic, finely chopped
- 4 scallions, finely chopped, plus more for serving
- ½ cup frozen peas, thawed
- 4 cups cauliflower rice
- 2 tbsp low-sodium soy sauce
- 2 tsp rice vinegar

- Kosher salt and pepper

Instructions:

1. Beat the chicken breast to an even thickness.
2. Heat 1 tbsp oil in a large skillet, over medium high heat.
3. Add chicken and cook 3-4 minutes per side or until golden brown.
4. Transfer to a cutting board and let cool for 5 minutes. Slice after cooled.
5. Add 1 tbsp oil to the skillet.
6. Add eggs and scramble for 1-2 minutes. Remove from the skillet and put aside.
7. In the skillet, cook bell pepper, carrot, and onion about 5 minutes or until tender.
8. Stir in garlic and cook for 1 minute.
9. Add peas and scallions and toss.
10. Add cauliflower, soy sauce, vinegar, salt and pepper. Toss.
11. Let cauliflower cook, without stirring, until it begins to brown.
12. Toss in sliced chicken and eggs.

Sheet Pan Steak

Total Time: 50 minutes

Serving Size: 4

Nutritional Facts:

> *calories: 464*
> *carbs: 26g*
> *fat: 22g*
> *protein: 42g*

Ingredients:

- 1 lb. small cremini mushrooms, trimmed and halved
- 1 ¼ lb. bunch broccolini, trimmed and cut into 2 inch lengths
- 4 cloves garlic, finely chopped
- 3 tbsp olive oil
- ¼ tsp red pepper flakes
- ¼ tsp. each kosher salt and pepper
- 2 1-inch thick New York strip steaks, trimmed of excess fat
- 1 15 oz. can low-sodium cannellini beans, rinsed

Instructions:

1. Preheat the oven to 450 degrees F.
2. Toss the mushrooms, broccolini, garlic, oil, red pepper flakes and salt and pepper until coated. Place in a single layer on a rimmed baking sheet.
3. Roast for 15 minutes.
4. Push the vegetable mixture to the edges of the pan. Place the steaks in the center of the pan.
5. Roast the steaks until desired doneness.
6. Allow to cool on a cutting board for 5 minutes before slicing.
7. While the steak is cooling, add beans to the vegetables in the baking dish and toss to combine. Return to the oven and roast for about 3 minutes, until beans are heated.
8. Plate the steak, beans, and vegetables, and enjoy.

* * *

Pork Tenderloin with Butternut Squash and Brussel Sprouts

Total Time: 50 minutes

Serving Size: 4

Nutritional Facts:

calories: 401
carbs: 25g
fat: 15g
protein: 44g

Ingredients:

- 1 ¾ lb. pork tenderloin, trimmed
- salt and pepper
- 3 tbsp canola oil
- 2 sprigs fresh thyme
- 2 cloves garlic, peeled
- 4 cups brussel sprouts, trimmed and halved
- 4 cups diced butternut squash

Instructions:

1. Preheat the oven to 400 degrees F.
2. Season pork with salt and pepper.
3. Heat oil over medium high heat in a large cast-iron skillet.
4. Add pork and sear until golden brown, about 8-12 minutes.
5. Remove from the skillet.
6. Add the remaining oil to the skillet. Add thyme and garlic and cook for one minute.
7. Add brussels sprouts, squash and a pinch of salt and pepper. Cook 4-6 minutes, stirring occasionally.
8. Place pork on top of the vegetables and place in the oven.
9. Roast 15-20 minutes, or until the thickest part of the tenderloin reaches 140 degrees F.
10. Carefully remove the pan from the oven. Allow to cool 5 minutes before slicing and serving.
11. Plate pork and vegetables. Serve with a side of greens tossed with balsamic vinaigrette.

* * *

Wild Cajun Spiced Salmon

Total Time: 30 minutes

Serving Size: 4

Nutritional Facts:

> *calories: 408*
> *carbs: 9g*
> *fat: 23g*
> *protein: 42g*

Ingredients:

- 1 ½ lb. wild Alaskan salmon fillet
- Sodium-free taco seasoning
- ½ head cauliflower, cut into florets
- 1 head broccoli, cut into florets
- 3 tbsp olive oil
- ½ tsp garlic powder
- 4 medium tomatoes, diced

Instructions:

1. Preheat the oven to 375 degrees F.
2. Mix taco seasoning with ½ cup water in a small bowl.
3. Place salmon in a baking dish. Pour taco seasoning mixture over fish.
4. Bake for 12-15 minutes.
5. While the salmon is baking, place the cauliflower and broccoli in a food processor.
6. Pulse into finely chopped.
7. Heat oil over medium heat in a large skillet. Add the riced cauliflower and broccoli. Sprinkle in garlic powder and cook, tossing, 5-6 minutes.
8. Plate the 'rice'; place salmon on top and top with tomatoes.

***

Pork Chops with Bloody Mary Tomato Salad

Total Time: 25 minutes

Serving Size: 4

Nutritional Facts:

calories: 400
carbs 8g
fat: 23g
protein: 39g

Ingredients:

- 2 tbsp olive oil
- 2 tbsp red wine vinegar
- 2 tsp Worcestershire sauce
- 2 tsp prepared horseradish, squeezed dry
- ½ tsp Tabasco
- ½ tsp celery seeds
- Kosher salt
- 1 pint cherry tomatoes, halved
- 2 celery stalks, very thinly sliced
- ½ small red onion, thinly sliced
- 4 small bone-in pork chops (1 inch thick)
- pepper

- ¼ cup finely chopped flat-leaf parsley
- 1 small head green-leaf lettuce, torn

Instructions:

1. Heat grill to medium high heat.
2. Mix together oil, vinegar, Worcestershire sauce, horseradish, Tabasco, celery seeds, and ¼ tsp salt in a large mixing bowl. Add tomato, celery, onion and toss until coated.
3. Salt and pepper the pork chops to taste, and grill 5-7 minutes per side.
4. Fold together the parsley and tomatoes; serve over pork chops and greens.
5. Serve with mashed cauliflower or potatoes.

* * *

BONUS MEAL IDEAS AND RECIPES

FASTING DAYS

If you are on a fasting diet which allows you to consume some calories, such as 5:2 or modified fasting for women, here are some great ideas to keep you full until your next meal. Don't forget to plan, and even prepare ahead. If you have these made and within easy reach, you are more likely to stick to the plan and not grab something you should not. Also, even though these are 'fasting meals', there is no harm in eating them during your eating window either.

Skin-Healthy Smoothie

This smoothie has enough healthy fats and fiber to keep you full, but also has antioxidants for your skin.

Serving Size: 1

Ingredients:

- Half an avocado
- A handful of kale
- 1 Tbsp flax seeds and/or chia seeds
- 1 cup non-dairy milk
- 1 serving of vanilla collagen protein supplement
- 1 date or 1/2 banana
- A sprinkle of cinnamon

Instructions:

1. Place all ingredients into a blender and blend until smooth.

* * *

Green Smoothie

Serving Size: 2

Ingredients:

- 1 banana
- ½ avocado
- 4 fists of spinach, black cabbage or formentino
- 2 squeezed oranges
- 1 cup of water
- 4 dates without stones
- 1 piece of grated ginger (the size of a garlic clove)

Instructions:

1. Blend all the ingredients for 30-60 seconds and enjoy!

* * *

Carrot Cake Smoothie

Serving Size: 1

Ingredients:

- 1 ½ cup of grated carrot
- 1 banana
- 3 spoons of walnuts
- 2 spoons of coconut milk
- 1 cup of water
- 1 spoon full of vegetable protein of your choice
- a pinch of coconut flakes
- a pinch of cinnamon
- 1 cup of ice

Instructions:

1. Place all ingredients in a blender and blend about 60 seconds, until smooth.

* * *

MEAL IDEAS

All of the following meal ideas were taken from the article "10 days of meal ideas for 5:2 fasting days", found on the Get the Gloss Website. As the title indicates, they are designed for people following the 5:2 method of intermittent fasting. These meal ideas will allow you to get through two fasting cycles, then you can mix and match to create more variety, as all food portions listed have calorie count as well. Remember that you can have 500 calories on your fasting days. These calories should be jammed packed with nutrients for all macronutrients, as the following meals are (Get The Gloss, 2017).

Fast Day Plan 1

Total calorie count: 525

Breakfast: *calories: 255*

Quaker Oats sachet of porridge (40g)

Dinner: *calories: 125*

Beetroot and feta salad

- beetroot (50g)
- feta (30g)
- spinach (60g)

- squeeze of lemon

Snack: *calories: 145*

Sliced apple with 1 tbsp of almond butter

Fast Day Plan 2

Total calorie count: 340

Breakfast: *calories: 145*

Sweet plums and yogurt

- 100g low fat natural yogurt
- 2 plums
- 1 tsp of honey

Dinner: *calories: 253*

Ryvita and tuna slices

- 2 x original Ryvita cracker breads
- tuna mayo (60g)
- rocket (70g) sprinkled on top
- cracked black pepper

Snack: *calories: 32*

Miso Soup

Fast Day Plan 3

Total calorie count: 478

Breakfast: *calories: 90*

Soft boiled egg and asparagus

- 1 egg
- 5 pieces of asparagus
- salt and pepper to season

Dinner: *calories: 328*

Turkey burgers with corn-on-the-cob

- minced turkey beaten with small egg, spring onion, garlic and chilli (111g)
- 1 x corn-on-the-cob

Snack: *calories: 60*

A few frozen grapes

Fast Day Plan 4

Total calorie count: 493

Breakfast: *calories: 228*

Packet of Belvita Breakfast Biscuits (muesli)

Dinner: *calories: 261*

Roasted vegetables with balsamic glaze

- ½ courgette, ½ aubergine, ½ butternut squash, ½ red pepper
- 1 tbsp balsamic vinegar
- squeeze of lemon

Snack: *calories: 4*

Harley's sugar-free jelly pot

Fast Day Plan 5

Total calorie count: 419

Breakfast: *calories: 160*

Spinach omelette

- 2 x eggs
- spinach leaves (60g)
- salt and pepper

Dinner: *calories: 175*

Hummus and crudites

- hummus (40g)
- a medium bowl full of carrots, cucumber, raw pepper

Snack: *calories: 84*

Edamame beans (60g) and rock salt

Fast Day Plan 6

Total calorie count: 452

Breakfast: *calories: 175*

Banana and low fat yogurt

- 100g low fat natural yogurt
- 1 x banana
- sprinkle of cinnamon

Dinner: *calories: 216*

Turkey breasts with wilted spinach

- 1 x turkey breast steak (125g)
- 1 cup of spinach, cooked and seasoned with salt

Snack: *calories: 59*

- 10g of popcorn

Fast Day Plan 7

Total calorie count: 452

Breakfast: *calories: 107*

Apple, carrot, and ginger smoothie

- 1 apple
- 1 carrot
- raw ginger

Dinner: *calories: 178*

Pita pizza

- Weight Watchers wholemeal pita
- 25g Extra Light Philadelphia cream cheese
- 1 tomato
- mixed herbs
- salt and pepper

Snack: *calories: 137*

- 100g blueberries and a handful of almonds

Fast Day Plan 8

Total calorie count: 489

Breakfast: *calories: 115*

Mixed berry bowl

- strawberries (100g)
- raspberries (100g)
- blueberries (100g)

Dinner: *calories: 314*

Harissa chicken with chargrilled vegetable couscous

- 1 x chicken breast (130g)
- 100g of vegetable couscous
- 1 tbsp harissa paste

Snack: *calories: 60*

Pistachios (around 10)

Fast Day Plan 9

Total calorie count: 424

Breakfast: *calories: 206*

Weight Watchers Blueberry Buttermilk Pancakes (3)

Dinner: *calories: 128*

Roasted red pepper and tomato soup with Ryvita cracker breads

- 2 x original Ryvita cracker breads
- ½ x red pepper, ½ x tomato, ½ onion, garlic clove, 1 tsp tomato puree, ½ tsp cumin, Oxo chicken, stock cube, ½ tsp balsamic vinegar, salt
- pepper to season

Snack: *calories: 90*

1 tbsp of pumpkin and sunflower seeds

Fast Day Plan 10

Total calorie count: 506

Breakfast: *calories: 190*

- Fruit and nut muesli (50g)

Dinner: *calories: 293*

Pesto salmon with curly kale

- salmon fillet (100g)
- 3 tsps of green pesto
- steamed kale, add black pepper (100g)

Snack: *calories: 23*

- 60g of stoned cherries

NON-FASTING DAYS

Non-fasting days do not mean cheat days or over-eat days. If you want to be successful while intermittent fasting, what you eat on your non-fasting days is just as important as what you put in your body on fasting days. You are supposed to eat as you normally would. However, many of us do not know what 'normal' eating should consist of. As a general rule, women need 2,000 and men need 2,700 calories a day (How Should I, 2014).

Keeping in mind that the average age is between 19-30, with women being just shy of 5'4" in height and 128 pounds, whereas for men it is 5'7" and 154 pounds and it is assumed the average is moderately active. Now ask yourself, how average are you? As we age, our calorie requirements fall, but our appetites do not (How Should I, 2014). Not to worry though, there are formulas to figure out how many calories you should be consuming each day. In fact, there are apps for that! These are the top recommended apps, according to Picard's article in Good Housekeeping (Picard, 2020). You can download one to find out your personal calorie needs and keep track of everything you consume that day to see if you are meeting or exceeding your daily caloric requirements:

- **Fitbit** While this app is mainly known for allowing you to count your steps and calories burned through exercise, it can also assist with calories required and calorie intake. You can enter calories from foods manually or simply scan their barcode. It can also break down your foods consumed into macronutrients. Don't have a fitbit? Don't worry, it can also work with your smartphone to track steps. This app is free for both Android and IOS users.

- **HealthyOut** This app is great for anyone who eats out or has dietary concerns and restrictions. It can suggest restaurants dishes that will not exceed your chosen meal count and break the meal into macronutrient percentages. It can also advise on low-carb, paleo, gluten free, and even "no salads" restaurants. This app is free for IOS users.

- **LoseIt** You get a personalized calorie budget based on your age, gender, weight, height. You can input your food by searching for the item, using the barcode scanner or even taking a picture of the meal to be evaluated! This app can be synced with other trackers for exercise tracking and with other members for support and accountability. Also has a premium version for even more personalized services. Available for Android and IOS devices.

- **MyFitnessPal** Perhaps this is the most popular app among the nutrition and exercise worlds. It has over five million foods stored, including portion sizes and protein content. This app can remember the food you've eaten in the past for easier entry and can even calculate calories of recipes from other sites. Extra, personalized features are available at a monthly premium.

- **Nutritionix Track** This app is recommended for its ease of use and transparency. It can track packaged food, restaurant meals, and fresh food. Great for eating a meal of mixed foods, such as takeout leftovers, with home cooked leftovers, and fresh ingredients. You can enter your food through a voice option as well. For an extra $5.99 a month, you have access to the Track Pro Coach Portal. IOS and Android apps available.

These are just some of the apps out there. By the time you read this list, there are sure to be many more available. Take the time to explore, ask questions and get recommendations, and see which one you feel will work best for you personally.

Eating too little on your non-fasting days can impair your weight loss journey as well. Undereating causes the release of cortisol, the stress hormone. Cortisol then increases insulin resistance, which causes the body to store fat, rather than burn it, which in turn, slows down weight loss. Under-eating can also slow down your metabolic rate and increase your hunger.

MEAL IDEAS

The following fourteen day meal plan comes from the article "14 day clean-eating meal plan : 2000 calories" composed by Registered Dietician Victoria Seaver M.S., as found on the Eating Well Website. Any food with an * at the end indicates that the recipe for that food is found at the end of the 14 day plan (Seaver, 2019).

Non-Fast Day Plan 1

Nutritional Facts:

> *calories: 1985*
> *carbohydrates: 240 g*
> *fat: 86 g*
> *protein: 82 g*

Breakfast

calories: 393

- 1 serving Muesli with Raspberries*
- 1 medium banana

A.M. Snack

calories: 216

- 1 medium orange
- 20 almonds

Lunch

calories: 550

- 4 cups White Bean & Veggie Salad*
- 1/4 cup hummus
- 8 seeded crackers

P.M. Snack

calories: 305

- 1 medium apple, sliced
- 2 tbsp. peanut butter

Dinner

calories: 420

- 4 cups (1 1/2 servings) Kale Salad with Beets & Wild Rice*
- 1 serving Balsamic-Dijon Chicken*

Evening Snack

calories: 101

- 1 medium pear, sliced and sprinkled with cinnamon

Non-Fast Day Plan 2

Nutritional Facts:

calories: 2003
carbs: 225g
fat: 90g
protein: 88g

Breakfast

calories: 542

- 2 servings Avocado-Egg Toast*

A.M. Snack

calories: 294

- 1 medium pear
- 25 almonds

Lunch

calories: 414

- 2 cups mixed greens
- 1/2 cup chopped cucumber
- 1/2 Balsamic-Dijon Chicken breast*, chopped
- 2 Tbsp. Lemon-Tahini Dressing*
- 2 Tbsp. sunflower seeds
- *Combine greens, cucumber and chicken and top with dressing and sunflower seeds.*
- 1 medium orange

P.M. Snack

calories: 201

- 1 medium banana
- 1 Tbsp. peanut butter

Dinner

calories: 552

- 1 serving cup Squash & Red Lentil Curry*
- 1 cup Easy Brown Rice*

Non-Fast Day Plan 3

Nutritional Facts:

> *calories: 2014*
> *carbs: 285g*
> *protein: 82g*
> *fat: 72g*

Breakfast

calories: 393

- 1 serving Muesli with Raspberries*
- 1 medium banana

A.M. Snack

calories: 294

- 1 medium pear
- 25 almonds

Lunch

calories: 537

- 1 serving cups Squash & Red Lentil Curry*
- 1/4 cup hummus
- 10 seeded crackers

P.M. Snack

305 calories: 305

- 1 medium apple, sliced
- 2 Tbsp. peanut butter

Dinner

calories: 495

- 1 serving Asian Tilapia with Stir-Fried Green Beans*
- 1 1/2 cup Easy Brown Rice*

Non-Fast Day Plan 4

Nutritional Facts:

> *calories: 1994*
> *carbs: 271g*
> *fat: 65g*
> *protein: 102g*

Breakfast

calories: 562

- 3/4 cup rolled oats, cooked in 1 1/2 cups milk
- 1 medium banana, chopped
- 2 tbsp. slivered almonds

Cook oats and top with banana, almonds and a pinch of cinnamon.

A.M. Snack

calories: 315

- 15 seeded crackers
- 1/4 cup hummus
- 2 medium carrots, cut into sticks

Lunch

calories: 420

- 1 serving Veggie & Hummus Sandwich*
- 1 medium apple

P.M. Snack

calories: 105

- 1 cup nonfat plain Greek yogurt
- 1 medium plum, chopped

Top yogurt with plum.

Dinner

calories: 432

- 1 serving Sheet-Pan Chicken & Brussels Sprouts*
- 1 1/2 cups mixed greens dressed with 2 Tbsp. Lemon-Tahini Dressing*

Evening Snack

calories: 101

- 1 medium pear, sliced and sprinkled with cinnamon

Non-Fast Day Plan 5

Nutritional Facts:

calories: 1993
carbs: 187g
fat: 104g
protein:94g

Breakfast

calories: 420

- 1 serving Peanut Butter-Banana Cinnamon Toast*
- 1 cup nonfat plain Greek yogurt
- 1 medium plum, chopped

Top yogurt with plum.

A.M. Snack

calories: 210

- 1 medium apple
- 15 almonds

Lunch

calories: 555

- 4 cups White Bean & Veggie Salad*
- 1 slice sprouted-grain bread topped with 1 oz. Cheddar cheese and toasted

P.M. Snack

calories: 265

- 15 seeded crackers
- 1/4 cup hummus

Dinner

calories: 543

- 1 serving Pork Chops with Garlicky Broccoli*

Non-Fast Day Plan 6

Nutritional Facts:

> *calories: 1993*
> *carbs: 240g*
> *fat: 87g*
> *protein: 80g*

Breakfast

calories: 521

- 3/4 cup rolled oats, cooked in 1 1/2 cups milk
- cup raspberries
- 2 tbsp. slivered almonds

Cook oats and top with raspberries, almonds and a pinch of cinnamon.

A.M. Snack

calories: 101

- 1 medium pear

Lunch

calories: 433

- 1 serving Veggie & Hummus Sandwich*
- 10 seeded crackers

P.M. Snack

calories: 305

- 1 medium apple, sliced
- 2 tbsp. peanut butter

Dinner

calories: 523

- 1 serving Cauliflower Rice-Stuffed Peppers*
- 2 cups mixed greens dressed with 2 Tbsp. Citrus Vinaigrette*

Evening Snack

calories: 110

- 1 cup Pineapple Nice Cream*

Non-Fast Day Plan 7

Nutritional Facts:

> *calories: 2015*
> *carbs: 255g*
> *fat: 92g*
> *protein: 61g*

Breakfast

calories: 338

- 2 cups Jason Mraz's Avocado Green Smoothie*
- 1 plum

A.M. Snack

calories: 315

- 1 medium banana
- 2 tbsp. peanut butter

Lunch

calories: 502

- 2 1/4 cup Tomato, Cucumber & White-Bean Salad with Basil Vinaigrette*
- 1 slice sprouted-grain bread topped with 1 oz. Cheddar cheese and toasted
- 1 medium orange

P.M. Snack

calories: 315

- 15 seeded crackers
- 1/4 cup hummus
- 2 medium carrots, cut into sticks

Dinner

calories: 545

- 2 cups Mexican Cabbage Soup*
- 2 cups No-Cook Black Bean Salad*

Non-Fast Day Plan 8

Nutritional Facts:

> *calories: 2005*
> *carbs: 216g*
> *fat 98g*
> *protein: 76g*

Breakfast

calories: 439

- 1 serving Scrambled Eggs with Vegetables*
- 1 medium pear

A.M. Snack

calories: 315

- 1 medium banana
- 2 tbsp. peanut butter

Lunch

calories: 433

- 1 serving Veggie & Hummus Sandwich*
- 10 seeded crackers

P.M. Snack

calories: 150

- 2 No-Sugar-Added Oatmeal Cookies*

Dinner

calories: 566

- 1 serving Greek Kale Salad with Quinoa & Chicken*
- 2 tbsp. crumbled feta cheese
- 2 tbsp. sunflower seeds
- 1 slice sprouted-grain bread, toasted and drizzled with 1 tsp. olive oil

Evening Snack

calories: 102

- 1 serving Broiled Mango*

Non-Fast Day Plan 9

Nutritional Facts:

calories: 1994
carbs: 236g
fat: 102g
protein: 62g

Breakfast

calories: 472

- 2 cups Jason Mraz's Avocado Green Smoothie*
- 1 slice sprouted-grain bread, toasted and topped with 2 tsp olive oil and a pinch each of salt & pepper

A.M. Snack

calories: 217

- 1 medium pear
- 15 almonds

Lunch

calories: 545

- 2 cups Mexican Cabbage Soup*
- 2 cup No-Cook Black Bean Salad*

P.M. Snack

calories: 92

- 3/4 cup Kiwi & Mango with Fresh Lime Zest

Dinner

calories: 519

- 1 cup riced cauliflower, heated
- 1 serving Soy-Lime Roasted Tofu*
- 2 cups Colorful Roasted Sheet-Pan Veggies*
- 2 tbsp. Citrus Vinaigrette*

Top riced cauliflower with tofu, veggies and drizzle with the vinaigrette.

Evening Snack

calories: 150

- 2 No-Sugar-Added Oatmeal Cookies*

Non-Fast Day Plan 10

Nutritional Facts:

calories: 1985
carbs: 236g
fat: 79g
protein: 96g

Breakfast

calories: 391

- 1 serving Peanut Butter-Banana Cinnamon Toast*
- 1 medium pear

A.M. Snack

calories: 271

- 1 hard-boiled egg seasoned with a pinch each salt & pepper
- 25 almonds

Lunch

calories: 434

- 1 serving Chicken & Apple Kale Wraps*
- 1 cup raspberries

P.M. Snack

calories: 261

- 10 seeded crackers
- 1/4 cup hummus
- 2 medium carrots, cut into sticks

Dinner

calories: 628

- 1 serving Panko-Crusted Pork Chops with Asian Slaw*
- 1 cup Easy Brown Rice*

Non-Fast Day Plan 11

Nutritional Facts:

> *calories: 2020*
> *carbs: 208g*
> *fat: 98g*
> *protein: 94g*

Breakfast

calories: 332

- 1 serving Avocado-Egg Toast
- 1 medium orange

A.M. Snack

calories: 265

- 15 seeded crackers
- 1/4 cup hummus

Lunch

calories: 508

- 1 serving Greek Kale Salad with Quinoa & Chicken
- 2 tbsp. crumbled feta cheese
- 2 tbsp. sunflower seeds
- 1 cup raspberries

Top salad with feta and sunflower seeds.

P.M. Snack

calories: 286

- 1 medium apple
- 2 tbsp. peanut butter

Dinner

calories: 478

- 1 serving Salmon & Asparagus with Lemon-Garlic Butter Sauce*
- 1 cup Basic Quinoa*

Evening Snack

calories: 150

- 2 No-Sugar-Added Oatmeal Cookies

Non-Fast Day Plan 12

Nutritional Facts:

calories: 2005
carbs: 201g
fat: 97g
protein: 96g

Breakfast

calories: 420

- 1 serving Peanut Butter-Banana Cinnamon Toast*
- 1 cup nonfat plain Greek yogurt
- 1 medium plum, chopped

Top yogurt with plum.

A.M. Snack

calories: 294

- 1 medium pear
- 25 almonds

Lunch

calories: 526

- 2 cups Mexican Cabbage Soup*
- 2 cups mixed greens
- 2 tbsp. Citrus Vinaigrette*
- 2 tbsp. sunflower seeds
- *Toss greens in vinaigrette. Top with sunflower seeds.*
- 1 medium orange

P.M. Snack

calories: 192

- 1 hard-boiled egg, seasoned with a pinch each of salt and pepper
- 1 oz. Cheddar cheese

Dinner

calories: 572

- 1 serving Spaghetti Squash & Meatballs*
- 1 slice sprouted-grain bread, toasted and drizzled with 2 tsp. olive oil.

Non-Fast Day Plan 13

Nutritional Facts:

calories: 2019
carbs: 236g
fat: 95g
protein: 85g

Breakfast

calories: 437

- 1 cup nonfat plain Greek yogurt
- 1 cup blueberries
- 1/2 cup muesli

A.M. Snack

315 calories

- 1 medium banana
- 2 tbsp. peanut butter

Lunch

calories: 426

- 1 serving Veggie & Hummus Sandwich*
- 1 medium pear

P.M. Snack

calories: 244

- 1 medium apple
- 2 No-Sugar-Added Oatmeal Cookies*

Dinner

calories: 596

- 1 serving Zucchini Noodles with Avocado Pesto & Shrimp*
- 2 cups mixed greens topped with 2 Tbsp. Citrus Vinaigrette*

Non-Fast Day Plan 14

Nutritional Facts:

calories: 2000
carbs: 201g
fat: 103g
protein: 84g

Breakfast

calories: 376

- 1 serving Avocado-Egg Toast*
- 1 medium banana

A.M. Snack

calories: 294

- 1 medium pear
- 25 almonds

Lunch

calories: 441

- 2 1/4 cup Tomato, Cucumber & White-Bean Salad with Basil Vinaigrette*
- 1 slice sprouted-grain bread topped with 1 oz. Cheddar cheese and toasted

P.M. Snack

calories: 261

- 10 seeded crackers
- 1/4 cup hummus
- 2 medium carrots, cut into sticks

Dinner

calories: 628

- 1 serving Fish with Coconut-Shallot Sauce*
- 1 cup Basic Quinoa*
- 2 cups mixed greens topped with 1 Tbsp. Citrus Vinaigrette*

Muesli with Raspberries

Prep Time: 5 mins

Serving Size: 1

Ingredients:

- ⅓ cup muesli
- 1 cup raspberries
- ¾ cup low-fat milk

Instructions:

1. Top muesli with raspberries and milk and enjoy!

White Bean & Veggie Salad

Prep Time: 10 mins

Serving Size: 1

Ingredients:

- 2 cups salad greens
- ¾ cup veggies of your choice (cucumber, tomatoes, etc.)
- ⅓ cup canned white beans
- ½ avocado
- 1 tbsp red-wine vinegar
- 2 tsp olive oil
- ¼ tsp kosher salt
- Freshly ground pepper

Instructions:

1. Tear salad greens into bite size pieces.
2. Chop veggies of choice.
3. Chop avocado.
4. Combine the above ingredients in a medium size bowl.
5. Pour vinegar, oil, salt and pepper on top.
6. Toss to combine and plate.

Kale Salad with Beets & Wild Rice

Prep time: 20 mins

Serving Size: 4

Ingredients:

- 1 large bunch lacinato or kale, stems trimmed and chopped (8 cups)
- 1 medium beet
- 1 cup cooked wild rice
- ⅓ cup sunflower seeds, toasted
- 5 tbsp lemon-Tahini Dressing*

Instructions:

1. Peel, slice, then chop beet.
2. Combine kale, beet, rice, and seeds in a large bowl
3. Add Dressing and toss.
4. Plate and enjoy!

* * *

Lemon-Tahini Dressing

Prep Time: 5 mins

Serving Size: 5

Ingredients:

- 3 tbsp lemon juice
- 2 tbsp water
- 2 tbsp tahini
- 1 small clove of garlic, minced
- ½ tsp salt
- ⅛ tsp cayenne pepper

Instructions:

1. Whisk all ingredients together in a small sized bowl until well blended and smooth.

* * *

Balsamic-Dijon Chicken

Prep Time: 4 hours, 30 mins

Serving Size: 4

Ingredients:

- 4 boneless skinless chicken breast halves
- ⅓ cup Dijon mustard
- 3 tbsp balsamic vinegar
- 2 cloves garlic, minced
- 2 tsp fresh thyme or basil - crushed (or ½ tsp dried)

Instructions:

1. Put chicken into a large resealable plastic bag and set aside.
2. Make the marinade: stir together mustard, vinegar, garlic and thyme in a small bowl until smooth.
3. Pour marinade over chicken and seal the bag.
4. Turn the bag several times to coat the chicken well.
5. Place the bag in a shallow baking dish and place in the refrigerator for 4-24 hours.
6. Turn the bad occasionally.
7. Remove the chicken from the bag, draining in and saving the marinade.

8. Place chicken on the chicken on the rack of an uncovered grill, heated to medium heat.

9. Grill for 7 minutes, brushing occasionally with saved marinade.

10. Turn chicken and brush again with marinade.

11. Grill for 5-8 minutes longer or tender and no longer pink (165 degrees F).

* * *

Avocado-Egg Toast

Prep Time: 5 mins

Serving Size: 1

Ingredients:

- ¼ avocado
- ¼ tsp ground pepper
- ⅛ tsp garlic powder
- 1 slice whole-wheat bread
- 1 large egg
- 1 tsp Sriracha (optional)
- 1 tbsp scallion, sliced (Optional)

Instructions:

1. Mash avocado with pepper and garlic powder in a small bowl.
2. Fry the egg to taste.
3. While the egg is frying, toast the bread.
4. Top toast with avocado and egg.
5. Top with Sriracha and scallion if desired

* * *

Squash & Red Lentil Curry

Prep Time: 40 mins

Servings: 5

Ingredients:

- 2 tbsp canola oil
- 1 ½ cup chopped onion
- 2 cloves garlic, minced
- 1 tablespoon minced ginger
- 2 tsp curry powder (or garam masala)
- 1 20 ounce package cubed peeled butternut squash
- 1 cup red lentils
- 1 cup chopped fresh tomato (or 1 15 oz can diced tomatoes, drained)
- 1 ½ tsp salt
- 4 cups water
- 1 14 oz can lite coconut milk
- 5 lime wedges

Instructions:

1. in a large pot, heat oil over medium high heat.
2. Add onion, garlic, ginger and curry powder.

3. Cook for 2-3 minutes, stirring often, until onions soften.

4. Add squash, lentils, tomato, and salt.

5. Cook and stir for 1 minute.

6. Add water.

7. Cover and over high heat, bring to a boil.

8. Reduce heat to simmer and cover.

9. Cook, stirring occasionally about 20 minutes until the squash is tender and the lentils are almost broken down.

10. Stir in milk and simmer for another minute or until heated through.

* * *

Easy Brown Rice

Prep Time: 1 hour

Serving Size: 6

Ingredients:

- 2 ½ cup water (or broth)
- 1 cup brown rice

Instructions:

1. In a medium saucepan, combine rice and water (or broth).
2. Bring to a boil.
3. Reduce heat to low and cover.
4. Simmer for 40-50 minutes until tender and most of the liquid is absorbed.
5. Let stand 5 minutes.
6. Fluff with a fork and serve.

* * *

Asian Tilapia with Stir-Fried Green Beans

Prep Time: 1 hour

Serving Size: 4

Ingredients:

- 4 5 oz fresh or frozen tilapia fillets
- ¼ cup reduced-sodium soy sauce
- 1 tsp toasted sesame oil
- 1 clove garlic, minced
- ¼ cup water
- 1 pound fresh green beans
- 2 tbsp water
- 1 tbsp canola oil
- non-stick cooking spray
- 1 tbsp sesame seeds, toasted
- 2 green onions, thinly sliced (¼ cup)

Instructions:

1. If fish is frozen, thaw.
2. Rinse fish, pat dry.
3. Place in a shallow baking dish.
4. Make marinade: whisk soy sauce, ginger, sesame oil, and garlic in a small sized bowl.

5. Pour marinade over fish and turn it to coat.

6. Cover with foil and let sit at room temperature for 20 minutes.

7. Drain fish. saving the marinade, add ¼ cup water to it.

8. Combine the beans and 2 tbsp of water in a large nonstick skillet.

9. Cook, covered for 5 minutes over medium heat. Stir occasionally.

10. Add oil. Continue to cook, uncovered for 5 minutes or until the beans are crisp, yet tender. Stir frequently.

11. Transfer to plate and cover.

12. Coat a second large skillet with non-stick spray. Heat over medium-high heat.

13. Add fish and cook, turning once, for 6-8 minutes or until fish flakes apart with a fork.

14. Sprinkle beans with sesame seeds and place fish on top.

15. With a paper towel, carefully wipe out the non-stick skillet. Add marinade.

16. Cook and stir for 1 minute over medium-high heat.

17. Strain marinade through a fine mesh sieve and pour over fish.

18. Sprinkle with green onions.

Veggie & Hummus Sandwich

Prep Time: 10 mins

Serving Size: 1

Ingredients:

- 2 slices of whole-grain bread
- 3 tbsp hummus
- ¼ avocado
- ½ cup mixed salad greens
- ¼ medium red bell pepper
- ¼ cup sliced cucumber
- ¼ cup shredded carrot

Instructions:

1. Mash the avocado
2. Spread one slice of bread with hummus, the other side with avocado.
3. Tear the salad greens into bite sized pieces and place on the bread.
4. Slice the bell pepper and place on bread.
5. Place the cucumber and carrot on the bread as well.
6. Slice in half and plate.

Garlic Hummus

Prep Time: 10 mins

Serving Size: 8

Ingredients:

- 1 15oz can of no salt added chickpeas
- ¼ cup tahini
- ¼ cup extra virgin olive oil
- ¼ cup lemon juice
- 1 clove garlic
- 1 tsp ground cumin
- ½ tsp chili powder
- ½ tsp salt

Instructions:

1. Drain chickpeas, keeping ¼ cup liquid.
2. Place chickpeas and liquid in the food processor.
3. Add the remaining ingredients.
4. Puree 2-3 minutes or until smooth.

Sheet-Pan Chicken & Brussel Sprouts

Prep Time: 35

Serving Size: 4

Ingredients:

- 1 pound sweet potatoes
- 2 tbsp extra virgin olive oil, divided
- ¾ tsp salt, divided
- ¾ ground pepper, divided
- 4 cups brussel sprouts, quartered
- 1 ¼ pound boneless, skinless chicken thighs, trimmed
- ½ teaspoon ground cumin
- ½ tsp dried thyme
- 3 tbsp sherry vinegar

Instructions:

1. Preheat the oven to 425 degrees F.
2. Peel and wedge the sweet potatoes.
3. Toss potatoes with 1 tbsp oil and ¼ tsp each salt and pepper.
4. Spread in a single layer on a rimmed baking sheet.
5. Cook for 15 minutes.

6. Remove from over. Do not turn the oven off.

7. Toss brussel sprouts with the remaining oil, ¼ tsp each salt and pepper.

8. Mix the brussel sprouts and potatoes together on the baking sheet.

9. Mix the cumin, thyme, and remaining ¼ tsp each of salt and pepper.

10. Sprinkle the spice mixture over the chicken.

11. Place chicken over the vegetables.

12. Bake for another 10-15 minutes or until the chicken is cooked and the vegetables are tender.

13. Once cooked, remove from the oven.

14. Remove chicken and place on a serving platter.

15. Place vegetables into a different serving dish and stir with the vinegar.

16. Serve chicken and vegetables together.

* * *

Peanut Butter-Banana Cinnamon Toast

Prep Time: 5 mins

Serving Size: 1

Ingredients:

- 1 slice whole-wheat bread
- 1 tbsp peanut butter
- 1 small banana
- Cinnamon to taste

Instructions:

1. Toast bread.
2. Slice the banana while bread is toasting.
3. Spread peanut butter on the toast.
4. Top with banana slices.
5. Sprinkle with cinnamon.

* * *

Pork Chops with Garlicky Broccoli

Prep Time: 30 mins

Serving Size: 4

Ingredients:

- 1 ½ pound broccoli with stems, trimmed and cut into spears
- 6 tbsp extra virgin olive oil, divided
- 1 cup panko breadcrumbs (preferably whole-wheat)
- ¼ cup grated Parmesan cheese (plus more for serving)
- ¼ cup whole-wheat flour
- 1 large egg
- 4 4oz boneless pork chops, trimmed
- ¾ tsp salt divided
- 1 tsp lemon juice
- 4 cloves garlic, thinly sliced
- ¼ tsp crushed red pepper
- 2 tbsp red-wine vinegar

Instructions:

1. Place the oven rack on the upper third of the oven.
2. Preheat the broiler to high setting.
3. Line a baking sheet with foil.
4. Toss 1 ½ tbsp oil with the broccoli and spread it on the lined baking sheet.
5. Boil for about 10 minutes, stirring once.
6. Remove from the oven and place in a bowl.
7. In a shallow bowl, mix the parmesan with the breadcrumbs.
8. In another shallow bowl, beat the egg slightly.
9. Place the flour in another shallow dish.
10. Sprinkle pork with ¼ tsp salt then dip in the flour, shaking off excess.
11. Then dip the floured pork into the egg, letting it drip.
12. Finally, coat the pork in the breadcrumb mixture.
13. In a large, non-stick skillet, heat 3 tbsp oil over medium-high heat.
14. Add pork and cook for about 6 minutes, turning midway through.
15. Remove from the skillet and place on a plate. Sprinkle with lemon juice. Cover with foil to keep warm.
16. With a paper towel, wipe the skillet.

17. Add 1 ½ tbsp oil, garlic, red pepper, and cook about 3 minutes over low heat. Stirring occasionally.
18. Remove from heat and stir in vinegar and ½ tsp salt.
19. Pour over broccoli and toss.
20. Serve the pork and broccoli with more parmesan, if desired.

* * *

Cauliflower Rice-Stuffed Peppers

Prep Time: 1 hours

Serving Size: 4

Ingredients:

- 4 large bell peppers
- 2 cups chopped cauliflower florets
- 2 tbsp extra-virgin Olive Oil, divided
- Pinch of salt, plus ½ tsp, divided
- Pinch ground pepper, plus ½ tsp, divided
- ½ cup chopped onion
- 1 pound lean ground beef
- 2 cloves garlic, minced.
- ½ tsp dried oregano
- 1 8 oz can no-salt-added tomato sauce
- ½ cup shredded part-skim mozzarella

Instructions:

1. Preheat the oven to 350 degrees F.
2. Slice the stem ends of the peppers.
3. Cut the flesh from the stem and chop.
4. Scoop the seeds from inside the peppers.

5. In a pot with a steamer basket, bring about an inch of water to a boil.

6. Place the peppers in the steamer basket and steam for about 3 minutes or until soft.

7. Remove peppers and set aside.

8. Place the cauliflower in a food processor. Pulse until it is in rice sized pieces.

9. Over medium heat, heat 1 tbsp of oil in a large skillet.

10. Add cauliflower rice and pinch of salt and pepper.

11. Stir softly and cook for about 3 minutes or until browned.

12. Remove from the skillet and place in a small bowl.

13. Using a paper towel, wipe out the skillet.

14. Add remaining 1 tbsp of oil, chopped pepper and onion.

15. Cook for about 3 minutes, stirring occasionally.

16. Add beef, garlic, oregano, and remaining ½ tsp each of salt and pepper.

17. Break up the beef with a wooden spoon as it cooks.

18. Cook about 5 minutes or until beef is no longer pink.

19. Ass tomato sauce and cauliflower rice. Stir just enough to coat.

20. Place peppers upright in an 8" baking dish.

21. Fill each pepper with 1 cup of cauliflower mixture.

22. Top each pepper with 2 tablespoons of cheese.

23. Bake for 20-25 minutes until heated through and cheese is melted.

* * *

Citrus Vinaigrette

Prep Time: 10 mins

Serving Size: 8

Ingredients:

- ½ small shallot, quartered
- 1 tsp orange zest
- ¼ cup orange juice
- 2 tbsp lemon juice
- 2 tsp Dijon mustard
- ½ tsp salt
- ½ tsp ground pepper
- ¼ cup extra-virgin olive oil
- ¼ cup canola or avocado oil

Instructions:

1. Place shallot, zest, juices, mustard, salt and pepper in a blender or food processor. Add oil and blend until smooth.

Pineapple Nice Cream

Total Prep Time: 5 mins / Servings: 6

Ingredients:

- 1 16 oz package frozen pineapple chunks
- 1 cup frozen mango chunks (or 1 large mango, peeled, seeded, and chopped)
- 1 tbsp lemon or lime juice

Instructions:

1. Place all ingredients into a food processor and blend until smooth and creamy.

* * *

Jason Mraz's Avocado Green Smoothie

Prep Time: 15 mins

Serving Size: 2

Ingredients:

- 1 ¼ cup cold unsweetened almond milk
- 1 ripe avocado
- 1 ripe banana
- 1 sweet apple, such as honeycrisp, sliced
- ½ large celery stalk, chopped
- 2 cups lightly packed kale leaves or spinach
- 1 1" piece of fresh peeled ginger
- 8 ice cubes

Instructions:

1. Place ingredients in the blender in the order listed and blend until smooth.

* * *

Tomato, Cucumber & White-Bean Salad with Basil Vinaigrette

Prep Time: 25 mins

Serving Size: 4

Ingredients:

- ½ cup packed fresh basil leaves
- ¼ cup extra virgin olive oil
- 3 tbsp red-wine vinegar
- 1 tbsp finely chopped shallot
- 2 tsp Dijon mustard
- 1 tsp honey
- ¼ tsp salt
- ¼ tsp ground pepper
- 10 cups mixed salad greens
- 1 15oz can low-sodium cannellini beans, rinsed
- 1 cup halved cherry or grape tomatoes.
- ½ cucumber, halved lengthwise and sliced (1 cup)

Instructions:

1. Make vinaigrette: Process basil, oil, vinegar, shallot, mustard, honey, salt and pepper in a food processor until smooth.
2. Place in a large bowl.
3. Add greens, beans, tomatoes and cucumber.
4. Toss and serve.

* * *

Mexican Cabbage Soup

Total Prep Time: 20 mins / Servings: 8

Ingredients:

- 2 tbsp extra virgin olive oil
- 2 cups chopped onions
- 1 cup chopped carrot
- 1 cup chopped celery
- 1 cup chopped poblano or green bell pepper
- 4 large cloves garlic, minced
- 8 cups sliced cabbage
- 1 tbsp tomato paste
- 1 tbsp minced chipotle chiles in adobo sauce
- 1 tsp ground cumin
- ½ tsp ground coriander
- 4 cup low-sodium vegetable broth or chicken broth
- 4 cups water
- 2 15 oz cans low-sodium pinto or black beans, rinsed
- ¾ tsp salt
- ½ cup chopped fresh cilantro, plus more for serving.
- 2 tbsp lime juice

Instructions:

1. In a large soup pot, heat oil over medium heat.
2. Add onion, carrot, celery, poblano, and garlic.
3. Cook 10-12 minutes, stirring frequently, until softened.
4. Add cabbage and cook for another 10 minutes or until softened.
5. Add tomato paste, chipotle, cumin and coriander.
6. Cook one additional minute, stirring.

* * *

No-Cook Black Bean Salad

Prep Time: 30 mins

Serving Size: 4

Ingredients:

- ½ cup thinly sliced red onion
- 1 medium ripe avocado, pitted and chopped
- ¼ cup cilantro leaves
- ¼ cup lime juice
- 2 tbsp extra virgin olive oil
- 1 clove garlic, minced
- ½ tsp salt
- 8 cups mixed salad greens
- 2 cups frozen corn, thawed and patted dry
- 1 pint grape tomatoes, halved
- 1 15 oz can black beans, rinsed

Instructions:

- In a medium bowl, cover onion with cold water.
- In a food processor, combine avocado, cilantro, lime juice, oil, garlic, and salt until smooth and creamy.

- In a large bowl combine greens, corn, tomatoes and beans. Drain the onions and add.
- Add the avocado dressing and mix until well coated.

* * *

Scrambled Eggs with Vegetables

Prep Time: 20 mins

Serving Size: 1

Ingredients:

- 2 tsp olive oil
- 1 cup chopped broccoli, asparagus and/or zucchini
- 1 small clove, minced
- ½ tsp minced fresh rosemary
- 2 large eggs
- 1 tbsp heavy cream
- ⅛ tsp salt
- ¼ tsp ground pepper
- 1 tbsp shredded Cheddar or Gouda Cheese

Instructions:

1. In a medium sized skillet, heat oil over medium low heat.
2. Add chopped vegetables.
3. Stirring often, cook until tender. 2-4 minutes.
4. Add garlic and rosemary. Stir while cooking for another minute.

5. In a small bowl, whisk eggs, with cream, salt and pepper.

6. Pour over cooked vegetables.

7. Stir until eggs are almost set.

8. Add cheese.

9. Turn off heat and let eggs sit until cheese is melted.

* * *

No Sugar Added Oatmeal Cookies

Prep Time: 1 hour, 15 mins

Serving Size: 15

Ingredients:

- 1 ½ cup quick cooking oats
- 1 cup oat flour
- ¾ tsp ground cinnamon
- ¼ tsp baking soda
- ¼ tsp salt
- 2 medium bananas, ripe and mashed
- 2 large eggs
- ¼ cup melted coconut oil or unsalted butter
- ¾ cup chopped dates or raisins
- ½ cup shredded unsweetened coconut
- 1 tsp vanilla extract

Instructions:

1. Preheat the oven to 350 degrees F.
2. Line a cookie sheet with parchment paper.
3. In a large bowl, combine oats, flour, cinnamon, baking soda, and salt.

4. In another bowl, whisk eggs, coconut oil, and vanilla. Mix in mashed bananas.

5. Add dry ingredients then the dates and coconut to the banana mixture and stir until well combined.

6. By the teaspoonful, roll the dough into balls and place on the baking sheet.

7. Press slightly with a fork.

8. Bake 15-17 minutes until lightly browned.

9. Cool on a wire rack before eating.

* * *

Greek Kale Salad with Quinoa & Chicken

Prep Time: 10 mins

Serving Size: 2

Ingredients:

- 4 cups chopped kale
- 1 ½ cups shredded cooked chicken
- 1 cup cooked quinoa
- ¼ cup sliced jarred roasted red peppers
- ¼ cup Greek salad dressing
- 1 oz crumbled feta cheese

Instructions:

1. In a large bowl, combine kale, chicken, quinoa and roasted peppers.
2. Add dressing and toss.
3. Plate and top with feta.

* * *

Broiled Mango

Prep Time: 20 mins

Serving Size: 2

Ingredients:

- 1 mango, peeled and sliced
- Lime wedges

Instructions:

1. Place the oven rack on the upper third of the over. Turn Boiler on.
2. Line a baking sheet with foil.
3. Arrange the mango on the pan.
4. Broil 8-10 minutes, until lightly browned in spots.
5. Plate and squeeze lime wedges over mango.

* * *

Soy-Lime Roasted Tofu

Prep Time: 1 hour, 35 mins

Serving Size: 4

Ingredients:

- 2 14 oz packages of extra-firm, water packed tofu, drained
- ⅔ cup reduced-sodium soy sauce
- ⅔ cup lime juice
- 6 tbsp toasted sesame oil

Instructions:

1. Pat tofu dry and cube.
2. In a large resealable bag, combine soy sauce, lime juice and oil. Add tofu to the bag and shake gently.
3. Place in the refrigerator for 1-4 hours. Gently tossing once or twice.
4. Preheat the oven to 450 degrees F.
5. Using a slotted spoon remove tofu from the bag.
6. Spread tofu on two large baking sheets, so that pieces are not touching.
7. Bake ~20 minutes, turning halfway or until golden brown.

Colorful Roasted Sheet-Pan Veggies

Prep Time: 45 mins

Serving Size: 8

Ingredients:

- 3 cups cubed butternut squash
- 3 tbsp extra virgin olive oil, divided
- 4 cups broccoli florets
- 2 red bell pepper, cut into squares
- 1 large red onion, cut into bite sized chunks
- 2 tsp Italian seasoning
- 1 tsp kosher salt
- ¼ tsp pepper
- 1 tbsp balsamic vinegar

Instructions:

1. Preheat the oven to 425 degrees F.
2. In a large bowl, toss the squash with 1 tbsp of oil
3. Spread on a baking sheet and bake for 10 minutes.
4. While squash is baking, toss broccoli, peppers, onions, seasonings, with the remaining 2 tbsp oil until well coated.

5. Remove the squash and add to vegetables in the bowl. Mix.

6. Use two baking sheets to spread vegetables evenly.

7. Bake, stirring twice for 17-20 minutes or until vegetables are tender.

8. Sprinkle with vinegar.

* * *

Chicken & Apple Kale Wraps

Prep Time: 10 mins

Serving Size: 1

Ingredients:

- 1 tbsp mayonnaise
- 1 tsp Dijon mustard
- 3 medium kale leaves
- 3 oz thinly sliced cooked chicken breast
- 6 thin red onion slices
- 1 firm apple, cut into 9 slices

Instructions:

1. In a small bowl, mix the mayonnaise and mustard.
2. Spread mixture on kale leaves.
3. Top each leaf with 1 oz chicken, 2 onion slices and 3 apple slices.
4. Roll each leaf into a wrap.

Panko-Crusted Pork Chops with Asian Slaw

Prep Time: 40 mins

Serving Size: 4

Ingredients:

- 3 tbsp miso, divided
- 1 large egg
- 1 tsp hot sauce
- ½ tsp ground pepper, divided
- ¾ cup whole wheat panko breadcrumbs
- 4 boneless pork chops, trimmed
- 3 tbsp rice vinegar
- 2 tbsp avocado oil
- 1 tbsp mayonnaise
- 1 tsp grated ginger
- ⅛ tsp salt
- 5 cups shredded cabbage
- 2 cups sliced snow peas
- 1 cup sliced red bell peppers
- 2 scallions, sliced

Instructions:

1. Preheat the oven to 450 degrees F.
2. Place a wire rack on a rimmed baking sheet.
3. Spray the rack with non-stick cooking spray.
4. In a shallow disk, whisk the miso, egg, hot sauce and ¼ tsp pepper.
5. Place panko in another shallow dish.
6. Dip each pork chop in egg, then panko. Make sure to dip both sides.
7. Coat both sides of chops with cooking spray and place on the wire rack.
8. Bake 15-18 minutes until cooked through.
9. Slaw: In a large bowl, whisk vinegar, oil, mayonnaise, ginger, salt, remaining miso and remaining pepper.
10. Add cabbage, peas, peppers and scallions. Mix well.
11. Serve pork chops and slaw together.

Basic Quinoa

Prep Time: 30mins

Serving Size: 6

Ingredients:

- 2 cups water or broth
- 1 cup quinoa

Instructions:

1. In a medium saucepan, combine water or broth and quinoa.
2. Bring to a boil,, then cover and reduce to a simmer.
3. Simmer for 15-20 or until tender and most of the liquid is absorbed.
4. Fluff with a fork and serve.

* * *

Salmon & Asparagus with Lemon-Garlic Butter Sauce

Prep Time: 25 mins

Serving Size: 4

Ingredients:

- 1 pound of center-cut salmon fillet, cut into 4 portions
- 1 pound fresh asparagus, trimmed
- ½ tsp salt
- ½ tsp ground pepper
- 3 tbsp butter
- 1 tbsp butter
- 1 tbsp extra virgin Olive oil
- ½ tbsp grated garlic
- 1 tsp grated lemon zest
- 1 tbsp lemon juice

Instructions:

1. Preheat the oven to 375 degrees F.
2. Spray a large rimmed baking sheet with non-stick cooking spray.
3. Place salmon and asparagus on different ends of the baking sheet.

4. Sprinkle it with salt and pepper.

5. In a small skillet, over medium heat, heat butter, oil, garlic, lemon zest and lemon juice.

6. When butter is melted, drizzle it over the salmon and asparagus.

7. Bake for 12-25 minutes, until the salmon is flaky and the asparagus is tender.

* * *

Spaghetti Squash & Meatballs

Prep Time: 45 mins

Serving Size: 4

Ingredients:

- 1 3-pound spaghetti squash
- 2 tbsp water
- 2 tbsp extra-virgin olive oil, divided
- ½ cup chopped fresh parsley, divided
- ½ cup finely shredded Parmesan cheese, divided
- 1 ¼ tsp Italian seasoning, divided
- ½ tsp onion powder
- ½ tsp salt, divided
- ½ tsp ground pepper
- 1 pound lean ground turkey
- 4 large cloves garlic, minced
- 1 28 oz can no salt added crushed tomatoes
- ¼-½ tsp crushed red pepper

Instructions:

1. Cut squash in half, lengthwise and scoop out the seeds.
2. In a microwave safe dish, place and inch or two of water.
3. Place squash face down in the pan.
4. Microwave on high for 10-15 minutes or until a fork can easily scrap the flesh.
5. Let the squash cool until it can be easily handled.
6. Using a fork, scrap the flesh out of the squash, using long strokes (creating noodles) and put aside.
7. In a large skillet, over medium-high, heat 1 tsp of oil.
8. Cook the squash, stirring occasionally, for 5-10 minutes or until moisture is evaporated.
9. Stir in ¼ cup parsley.
10. Remove from heat, cover.
11. In a medium bowl, mix together ¼ cup parsley, ¼ cup Parmesan, ½ tsp Italian seasoning, onion powder, ¼ tsp salt and pepper.
12. Fold turkey into mixture until just combined.
13. Form into 12 meatballs, about 2 tbsp each.
14. In a large non-stick skillet, over medium heat, add 1 tbsp of oil, then meatballs.

15. Cook over medium heat, turning occasionally for 4-6 minutes or until browned.

16. Push to the side of the pan.

17. Add garlic and toss in the pan for 1 minute.

18. Add tomatoes, red pepper, Italian seasoning, and salt.

19. Stir until meatballs are coated.

20. Cover and simmer for 10-12 minutes, until meatballs are cooked.

21. Serve by placing quash on a plate, then meatballs and sauce. Sprinkle the ¼ cup Parmesan.

* * *

Zucchini Noodles with Avocado Pesto & Shrimp

Prep Time: 35 mins

Serving Size: 4

Ingredients:

- 5-6 medium zucchini, trimmed
- ¾ tsp salt, divided
- 1 avocado, ripe
- 1 cup poached fresh basil leaves
- ¼ cup unsalted shelled pistachios
- 2 tbsp lemon juice
- ¼ tsp ground pepper
- ¼ cup extra virgin olive oil plus 2 tbsp, divided
- 3 cloves garlic, minced
- 1 pound raw shrimp (21-25 count), peeled and deveined.
- 1-2 tsp Old Bay seasoning

Instructions:

1. Cut the zucchini lengthwise using spiral vegetable slices or a vegetable peeler to create long thin strips.
2. Stop when you reach the seeds.

3. Place zucchini noodles in a colander and toss with ½ tsp salt.

4. Let drain for 15-30 minutes.

5. Squeeze out any moisture.

6. In a food processor, combine avocado, basil, pistachios, lemon juice, pepper and ¼ tsp salt. Pulse until chopped fine.

7. Add ¼ cup oil and process until smooth.

8. Place a large skillet over medium-high heat and add 1 tbsp oil.

9. Add garlic, toss in oil for 30 seconds.

10. Add shrimp and Old Bay.

11. Cook for 3-4 minutes, stirring occasionally, until shrimp is almost cooked through.

12. Remove from heat and place in a large bowl

13. Add 1 tbsp oil to the skillet and add zucchini noodles.

14. Toss for about 3 minutes, until hot.

15. Add to shrimp.

16. Add pesto.

17. Toss all until combined.

Fish with Coconut-Shallot Sauce

Prep Time: 30 mins

Servings: 4

Ingredients:

- 3 cloves garlic, chopped
- ¾ tsp kosher salad, divided
- 2 tbsp extra virgin olive oil, divided
- 2 tbsp chopped fresh thyme (2 tsp dried)
- ¼ tsp ground pepper
- 1 ¼ pounds mahi-mahi, red snapper or grouper, skinned and cut into 4 portions
- 2 tbsp finely chopped shallot
- 1 cup lite coconut milk
- ¼ cup unsweetened coconut chips, toasted
- Lime wedges for serving

Instructions:

1. Place the rack in the upper third of the oven. Line a baking sheet with foil and spray with cooking spray.
2. Turn over broiler to high

3. Using a fork, mash together the garlic and ½ tsp salt, making a paste.

4. Mix paste with 1 tbsp oil, thyme, and ¼ tsp pepper

5. Place fish in a baking pan and spread paste on top.

6. In a medium skillet, over medium heat, heat 1 tbsp oil.

7. Add shallot and stir for 30 seconds.

8. Add coconut milk, increase heat to medium high, to bring milk to a simmer.

9. Reduce heat to medium low and simmer for about 6 minutes or until only ¾ cup milk mixture remains.

10. Add ¼ tsp salt and pepper.

11. Broil fish 6-8 minutes or until cooked through.

12. Plate and spoon sauce on top.

13. Sprinkle with coconut and serve with lime

PLEASE REVIEW

I certainly hope that you have found the information in *The Fasting Facts* interesting and helpful to you on your journey toward a healthier lifestyle. Please leave a review as to the ease and helpfulness of the information found within. Your honesty will allow me to better meet your needs and preferences in the future.

REFERENCES

5 Things You Need To Know About Intermittent Fasting And Breast Cancer. (n.d.). Rethink Breast Cancer. Retrieved February 26, 2021, from https://rethinkbreastcancer.com/5-things-you-need-to-know-about-intermittent-fasting-and-breast-cancer/

7 Different Types of Fasting Explained. (2018, September 13). 131 Method. https://blog.131method.com/different-types-of-fasting-explpained/

Abbate, E. (n.d.). *Intermittent Versus Time-Restricted: Which Fasting Is Best?* Spartan Race. Retrieved February 26, 2021, from https://www.spartan.com/blogs/unbreakable-nutrition/intermittent-fasting-schedule-vs-trf

American Heart Association. (2010). *Understanding Blood Pressure Readings.* Www.heart.org. https://www.heart.

org/en/health-topics/high-blood-pressure/understanding-blood-pressure-readings

Barna, M. (2019, January 1). *The Science Behind Fasting Diets*. Discover Magazine. https://www.discovermagazine.com/health/fasting-may-be-more-than-a-fad-diet

Berger, M. (2019, August 22). *How Intermittent Fasting Can Help Lower Inflammation*. Healthline; Healthline Media. https://www.healthline.com/health-news/fasting-can-help-ease-inflammation-in-the-body

Bjarnadottir, A., & Kubala, J. (2020, August 4). *Alternate-Day Fasting*. Healthline. https://www.healthline.com/nutrition/alternate-day-fasting-guide

Bradley, S., & Miller, K. (2021, January 15). *These Intermittent Fasting Apps Make It *So* Simple To Stay On Track*. Women's Health. https://www.womenshealthmag.com/weight-loss/g29554400/intermittent-fasting-apps/

Breus, M. (2019, April 11). *What Is Intermittent Fasting, and Will It Help Your Sleep?* Psychology Today. https://www.psychologytoday.com/ca/blog/sleep-newzzz/201904/what-is-intermittent-fasting-and-will-it-help-your-sleep#:~:text=The%20timing%20and%20duration%20of

Chronic stress puts your health at risk. (2019, March 19). Mayo Clinic. https://www.mayoclinic.org/healthy-lifestyle/

stress-management/in-depth/stress/art-
20046037#:~:text=Cortisol%2C%20the%20prima-
ry%20stress%20hormone

Collier, R. (2013). Intermittent fasting: the science of going without. *Canadian Medical Association Journal, 185*(9), E363–E364. https://doi.org/10.1503/cmaj.109-4451

Cording, J. (2020, October 28). What Is the Fasting Mimicking Diet and Is It Healthy? *Shape*. https://www.shape.com/healthy-eating/diets/fasting-mimicking-diet

Coyle, D. (2018, July 22). *Intermittent Fasting For Women: A Beginner's Guide*. Healthline. https://www.healthline.com/nutrition/intermittent-fasting-for-women#health-benefits

DeSantis, A. (2020, February 1). *Intermittent fasting and blood pressure*. Delicious Living. https://www.deliciousliving.com/health/intermittent-fasting-and-blood-pressure/

Dieting | nutrition | Britannica. (2019). In *Encyclopædia Britannica*. https://www.britannica.com/science/dieting

Editor. (2017, October 27). *Fasting may change the body's hunger response - here's what to do about it*. Diabetes. https://www.diabetes.co.uk/in-depth/fasting-may-change-bodys-hunger-response-heres/

Eenfeldt, A. (2020, December 16). *How to Normalize Your Blood Pressure Naturally*. Diet Doctor. https://www.dietdoctor.com/blood-pressure

Eknoyan, G. (2006). A History of Obesity, or How What Was Good Became Ugly and Then Bad. *Advances in Chronic Kidney Disease, 13*(4), 421–427. https://doi.org/10.1053/j.ackd.2006.07.002

English, N. (2019, April 11). *Does Intermittent Fasting Affect Women Differently Than Men?* BarBend. https://barbend.com/intermittent-fasting-women/

Fast Fix: Does Intermittent Fasting Help Your Skin? (n.d.). MirraSkincare. Retrieved February 25, 2021, from https://inthemirra.com/blogs/news/does-intermittent-fasting-help-your-skin#:~:text=Fasting%20Can%20Regulate%20Blood%20Glucose%20Levels&text=Just%20to%20refresh%20you%3A%20collagen

Fasting. (2021). In *Encyclopædia Britannica*. https://www.britannica.com/topic/fasting

Fatty Liver Disease: Risk Factors, Symptoms, Types & Prevention. (2020, July 31). Cleveland Clinic. https://my.clevelandclinic.org/health/diseases/15831-fatty-liver-disease

Fung, D. J. (2015, April 11). *Fasting - A History*. The Fasting Method. https://thefastingmethod.com/fasting-a-history-part-i/

Fung, J. (2016a, September 19). *Short fasting regimens – less than 24 hours*. Diet Doctor. https://www.dietdoctor.com/short-fasting-regimens

Fung, J. (2016b, October 3). *Longer Fasting Regimens – 24 Hours or More*. Diet Doctor. https://www.dietdoctor.com/longer-fasting-regimens#risks

Fung, J. (2016c, October 5). *How to Renew Your Body: Fasting and Autophagy*. Diet Doctor. https://www.dietdoctor.com/renew-body-fasting-autophagy

Fung, J. (2016d, November 6). *Fasting and cholesterol*. Diet Doctor. https://www.dietdoctor.com/fasting-and-cholesterol

Fung, J. (2019, April 25). *Diet Doctor*. Diet Doctor. https://www.dietdoctor.com/intermittent-fasting

Get The Gloss. (2017). *10 meal plan ideas for 5:2 fast days*. Get the Gloss. https://www.getthegloss.com/article/10-days-of-meal-ideas-for-5-2-fasting-days

Graeme, C. (2019, June 26). *Leangains: The Best Intermittent Fasting for Gaining Muscle?* BarBend. https://barbend.com/leangains/

Greenleatherr. (2019). *Dry Fasting : Guide to Miracle of Fasting - Healing the Body with Auophagy, Clearing the Mind, Energizing the Spirit, Weight Loss and Anti-aging.*

Gunners, K. (2020, September 25). *How Intermittent Fasting Can Help You Lose Weight.* Healthline. https://www.healthline.com/nutrition/intermittent-fasting-and-weight-loss#hormonal-effects

Hargrove, J. (2006, November 12). *Confusion About Calories Is Nothing New, Professor Finds.* ScienceDaily. https://www.sciencedaily.com/releases/2006/11/061120060301.htm#:~:text=A%20popular%20early%20nutrition%20text

Health, T. E. of W. (2020, January 30). *Need An Intermittent Fasting Meal Plan? Here's Your 7-Day Brunch And Dinner Plan To Break Your Fast.* Women's Health. https://www.womenshealthmag.com/weight-loss/a30658778/intermittent-fasting-meal-plan-men-s-health/

Heffernan, C. (2016, May 5). *The History of Calorie Counting.* Physical Culture Study. https://physicalculturestudy.com/2016/05/05/the-history-of-calorie-counting/

Horowitz, M. (2015, August 17). *Can intermittent fasting improve mood?* National Elf Service. https://www.

nationalelfservice.net/mental-health/depression/can-intermittent-fasting-improve-mood/

How should I eat on my non-fasting days? | FastDay Intermittent Fasting. (2014, April 4). FastDay.com | Lose Weight with the 5:2 Fast Diet. https://www.fastday.com/fasting/troubleshooting-and-myth-busting/im-fasting-but-not-loosing-weight-how-should-i-eat-on-my-non-fasting-days/#google_vignette

Intermittent Fasting: Women vs. Men | ISSA. (n.d.). Www.issaonline.com. Retrieved February 26, 2021, from https://www.issaonline.com/blog/index.cfm/2018/this-hot-diet-trend-is-not-recommended-for-women#:~:text=Overall%2C%20men%20tend%20to%20do

Kubala, J. (2019, January 29). *ProLon Fasting Mimicking Diet Review: Does It Work for Weight Loss?* Healthline. https://www.healthline.com/nutrition/fasting-mimicking-diet

Leonard, J. (2020, April 16). *7 ways to do intermittent fasting: Best methods and quick tips*. Www.medicalnewstoday.com. https://www.medicalnewstoday.com/articles/322293

Lindberg, S. (2020, September 1). *How to Exercise Safely During Intermittent Fasting*. Healthline. https://www.

healthline.com/health/how-to-exercise-safely-intermittent-fasting

Marshall, L. (n.d.). *Behind the Intermittent Fasting Fad*. WebMD. https://www.webmd.com/diet/news/20200624/behind-the-intermittent-fasting-fad

Mawer, R. (2019, September 23). *11 Ways to Boost Human Growth Hormone (HGH) Naturally*. Healthline; Healthline Media. https://www.healthline.com/nutrition/11-ways-to-increase-hgh

McKnight, X. (2018). *Intermittent Fasting: Learn How to Eat the Foods you Love and Still Lose Five to Ten Pounds in Less Than 30 Days. Proven Scientific Weight Loss for Serious Results.*

Metabolic syndrome - Symptoms and causes. (2019, March 14). Mayo Clinic. https://www.mayoclinic.org/diseases-conditions/metabolic-syndrome/symptoms-causes/syc-20351916#:~:text=Metabolic%20syndrome%20is%20a%20cluster

Muszalski, C. (2019, March 19). *16:8 Intermittent Fasting | Benefits & How to Do It Properly*. MYPROTEIN™. https://www.myprotein.com/thezone/nutrition/intermittent-fasting-lean-gains-168/

Newman, T. (2017, October 19). *How intermittent fasting can increase weight loss*. Www.medicalnewstoday.com. https://www.medicalnewstoday.com/articles/319791

Oberg, E. (n.d.). *Fasting Diet Benefits, Health Effects & Weight Loss*. MedicineNet. Retrieved February 25, 2021, from https://www.medicinenet.com/fasting_diets/article.htm

Orlando, A. (2020, January 2). *Do Men Lose Weight More Easily Than Women?* Discover Magazine. https://www.discovermagazine.com/health/do-men-lose-weight-more-easily-than-women

Panoff, L. (2019, September 26). *What Breaks a Fast? Foods, Drinks, and Supplements*. Healthline. https://www.healthline.com/nutrition/what-breaks-a-fast#fast-friendly-foods

Petre, A. (2016, November 14). *The 12 Best Foods to Boost Your Metabolism*. Healthline. https://www.healthline.com/nutrition/metabolism-boosting-foods#TOC_TITLE_HDR_5

Picard, C. (2020, October 12). *These Are Calorie Counting Apps That Can Actually Help You Lose Weight, According to Nutritionists*. Good Housekeeping. https://www.goodhousekeeping.com/health-products/g28246667/best-calorie-counting-apps/

Pilon, B. (2018, March 24). *Brad Pilon's "Eat Blog Eat" – Eat Stop Eat | Intermittent fasting | Weight Loss | The pursuit of happiness.* Bradpilon.com. https://bradpilon.com/

Raman, R. (2017, October 22). *Water Fasting: Benefits and Dangers.* Healthline; Healthline Media. https://www.healthline.com/nutrition/water-fasting

Related Conditions. (n.d.). Obesity Action Coalition. https://www.obesityaction.org/get-educated/related-conditions/

Richter, A. (2020, October 22). *The Ketogenic Diet: A Detailed Beginner's Guide to Keto.* Healthline. https://www.healthline.com/nutrition/ketogenic-diet-101#diet-types

Rios, E. (2017). *Fasting; Intermittent Fasting and Body-building.*

Santos-Longhurst, A. (2018, July 27). *Chronic Inflammation: Definition, Symptoms, Causes, and Treatment.* Healthline. https://www.healthline.com/health/chronic-inflammation#causes

Schabron, D. (2020, February 9). *Smoothie Recipes For Intermittent Fasting.* Intermittent Fasting Insight. https://

intermittentfastinginsight.com/smoothie-recipes-for-intermittent-fasting/

Scher, B. (2021, January 20). *What You Need to Know About OMAD*. Diet Doctor. https://www.dietdoctor.com/intermittent-fasting/omad

Schwartz, M. (2020, September 24). *Here's How to Fast for a Healthier Gut*. Health.com. https://www.health.com/nutrition/how-to-fast-healthy-gut

Seaver, V. (2019, June 25). *14-Day Clean-Eating Meal Plan: 2,000 Calories*. EatingWell. https://www.eatingwell.com/article/289076/14-day-clean-eating-meal-plan-2000-calories/

Shortsleeve, C. (2020, February 21). *Try it: fasting-mimicking*. Furthermore from Equinox. https://furthermore.equinox.com/articles/2020/02/fasting-mimicking-diet

Shulman, S. (2019, September 10). *Here's Exactly What Happens to Your Body When You Skip a Meal*. Prevention. https://www.prevention.com/weight-loss/a20470631/effects-of-skipping-meals/

Sinke, D. (n.d.). *A Complete Guide to Dry Fasting: How to start + Benefits*. 21 Day Hero. Retrieved February 25, 2021, from https://21dayhero.com/complete-guide-to-dry-fasting/

Sorenson, A. (2019). *The Science of intermittent fasting: Why Intermittent Fasting Works and How to do it the Right Way.*

The Full History of Juicing: Is it Just a Trend? - Well Pared | Billings, MT. (2017, November 27). Well Pared. https://wellpared.com/full-history-juicing-not-trend/

West, H. (2016, June 7). *Counting Calories 101: How to Count Calories to Lose Weight.* Healthline. https://www. healthline.com/nutrition/counting-calories-101#TOC_TITLE_HDR_9

What You Should Know Before You Start A Weight-loss Plan. (2020, May 27). Familydoctor.org. https:// familydoctor.org/what-you-should-know-before-you-start-a-weight-loss-plan/

Withworth, G. (2018, September 21). *Juice cleanse: Benefits, risks, and effects.* Www.medicalnewstoday.com. https://www.medicalnewstoday.com/articles/323136#potential-risks

Wnuk, A. (2018). *How Does Fasting Affect the Brain?* Brainfacts.org. https://www.brainfacts.org/thinking-sensing-and-behaving/diet-and-lifestyle/2018/how-does-fasting-affect-the-brain-071318

Wong, C. (2021, January 16). *What Is a Juice Cleanse?* Verywell Fit. https://www.verywellfit.com/juice-cleanse-89120